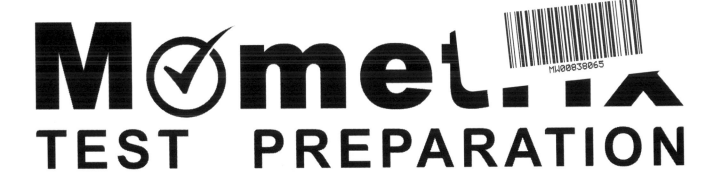

CCT

Exam Secrets
Study Guide

DEAR FUTURE EXAM SUCCESS STORY

First of all, **THANK YOU** for purchasing Mometrix study materials!

Second, congratulations! You are one of the few determined test-takers who are committed to doing whatever it takes to excel on your exam. **You have come to the right place.** We developed these study materials with one goal in mind: to deliver you the information you need in a format that's concise and easy to use.

In addition to optimizing your guide for the content of the test, we've outlined our recommended steps for breaking down the preparation process into small, attainable goals so you can make sure you stay on track.

We've also analyzed the entire test-taking process, identifying the most common pitfalls and showing how you can overcome them and be ready for any curveball the test throws you.

Standardized testing is one of the biggest obstacles on your road to success, which only increases the importance of doing well in the high-pressure, high-stakes environment of test day. Your results on this test could have a significant impact on your future, and this guide provides the information and practical advice to help you achieve your full potential on test day.

Your success is our success

We would love to hear from you! If you would like to share the story of your exam success or if you have any questions or comments in regard to our products, please contact us at **800-673-8175** or **support@mometrix.com**.

Thanks again for your business and we wish you continued success!

Sincerely,
The Mometrix Test Preparation Team

> **Need more help? Check out our flashcards at:**
> **http://MometrixFlashcards.com/CCT**

TABLE OF CONTENTS

Introduction

Thank you for purchasing this resource! You have made the choice to prepare yourself for a test that could have a huge impact on your future, and this guide is designed to help you be fully ready for test day. Obviously, it's important to have a solid understanding of the test material, but you also need to be prepared for the unique environment and stressors of the test, so that you can perform to the best of your abilities.

For this purpose, the first section that appears in this guide is the **Secret Keys**. We've devoted countless hours to meticulously researching what works and what doesn't, and we've boiled down our findings to the five most impactful steps you can take to improve your performance on the test. We start at the beginning with study planning and move through the preparation process, all the way to the testing strategies that will help you get the most out of what you know when you're finally sitting in front of the test.

We recommend that you start preparing for your test as far in advance as possible. However, if you've bought this guide as a last-minute study resource and only have a few days before your test, we recommend that you skip over the first two Secret Keys since they address a long-term study plan.

If you struggle with **test anxiety**, we strongly encourage you to check out our recommendations for how you can overcome it. Test anxiety is a formidable foe, but it can be beaten, and we want to make sure you have the tools you need to defeat it.

Secret Key 1: Plan Big, Study Small

There's a lot riding on your performance. If you want to ace this test, you're going to need to keep your skills sharp and the material fresh in your mind. You need a plan that lets you review everything you need to know while still fitting in your schedule. We'll break this strategy down into three categories.

Information Organization

Start with the information you already have: the official test outline. From this, you can make a complete list of all the concepts you need to cover before the test. Organize these concepts into groups that can be studied together, and create a list of any related vocabulary you need to learn so you can brush up on any difficult terms. You'll want to keep this vocabulary list handy once you actually start studying since you may need to add to it along the way.

Time Management

Once you have your set of study concepts, decide how to spread them out over the time you have left before the test. Break your study plan into small, clear goals so you have a manageable task for each day and know exactly what you're doing. Then just focus on one small step at a time. When you manage your time this way, you don't need to spend hours at a time studying. Studying a small block of content for a short period each day helps you retain information better and avoid stressing over how much you have left to do. You can relax knowing that you have a plan to cover everything in time. In order for this strategy to be effective though, you have to start studying early and stick to your schedule. Avoid the exhaustion and futility that comes from last-minute cramming!

Study Environment

The environment you study in has a big impact on your learning. Studying in a coffee shop, while probably more enjoyable, is not likely to be as fruitful as studying in a quiet room. It's important to keep distractions to a minimum. You're only planning to study for a short block of time, so make the most of it. Don't pause to check your phone or get up to find a snack. It's also important to **avoid multitasking**. Research has consistently shown that multitasking will make your studying dramatically less effective. Your study area should also be comfortable and well-lit so you don't have the distraction of straining your eyes or sitting on an uncomfortable chair.

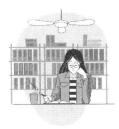

The time of day you study is also important. You want to be rested and alert. Don't wait until just before bedtime. Study when you'll be most likely to comprehend and remember. Even better, if you know what time of day your test will be, set that time aside for study. That way your brain will be used to working on that subject at that specific time and you'll have a better chance of recalling information.

Finally, it can be helpful to team up with others who are studying for the same test. Your actual studying should be done in as isolated an environment as possible, but the work of organizing the information and setting up the study plan can be divided up. In between study sessions, you can discuss with your teammates the concepts that you're all studying and quiz each other on the details. Just be sure that your teammates are as serious about the test as you are. If you find that your study time is being replaced with social time, you might need to find a new team.

Secret Key 2: Make Your Studying Count

You're devoting a lot of time and effort to preparing for this test, so you want to be absolutely certain it will pay off. This means doing more than just reading the content and hoping you can remember it on test day. It's important to make every minute of study count. There are two main areas you can focus on to make your studying count.

Retention

It doesn't matter how much time you study if you can't remember the material. You need to make sure you are retaining the concepts. To check your retention of the information you're learning, try recalling it at later times with minimal prompting. Try carrying around flashcards and glance at one or two from time to time or ask a friend who's also studying for the test to quiz you.

To enhance your retention, look for ways to put the information into practice so that you can apply it rather than simply recalling it. If you're using the information in practical ways, it will be much easier to remember. Similarly, it helps to solidify a concept in your mind if you're not only reading it to yourself but also explaining it to someone else. Ask a friend to let you teach them about a concept you're a little shaky on (or speak aloud to an imaginary audience if necessary). As you try to summarize, define, give examples, and answer your friend's questions, you'll understand the concepts better and they will stay with you longer. Finally, step back for a big picture view and ask yourself how each piece of information fits with the whole subject. When you link the different concepts together and see them working together as a whole, it's easier to remember the individual components.

Finally, practice showing your work on any multi-step problems, even if you're just studying. Writing out each step you take to solve a problem will help solidify the process in your mind, and you'll be more likely to remember it during the test.

Modality

Modality simply refers to the means or method by which you study. Choosing a study modality that fits your own individual learning style is crucial. No two people learn best in exactly the same way, so it's important to know your strengths and use them to your advantage.

4

For example, if you learn best by visualization, focus on visualizing a concept in your mind and draw an image or a diagram. Try color-coding your notes, illustrating them, or creating symbols that will trigger your mind to recall a learned concept. If you learn best by hearing or discussing information, find a study partner who learns the same way or read aloud to yourself. Think about how to put the information in your own words. Imagine that you are giving a lecture on the topic and record yourself so you can listen to it later.

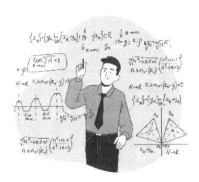

For any learning style, flashcards can be helpful. Organize the information so you can take advantage of spare moments to review. Underline key words or phrases. Use different colors for different categories. Mnemonic devices (such as creating a short list in which every item starts with the same letter) can also help with retention. Find what works best for you and use it to store the information in your mind most effectively and easily.

5

Secret Key 3: Practice the Right Way

Your success on test day depends not only on how many hours you put into preparing, but also on whether you prepared the right way. It's good to check along the way to see if your studying is paying off. One of the most effective ways to do this is by taking practice tests to evaluate your progress. Practice tests are useful because they show exactly where you need to improve. Every time you take a practice test, pay special attention to these three groups of questions:

- The questions you got wrong
- The questions you had to guess on, even if you guessed right
- The questions you found difficult or slow to work through

This will show you exactly what your weak areas are, and where you need to devote more study time. Ask yourself why each of these questions gave you trouble. Was it because you didn't understand the material? Was it because you didn't remember the vocabulary? Do you need more repetitions on this type of question to build speed and confidence? Dig into those questions and figure out how you can strengthen your weak areas as you go back to review the material.

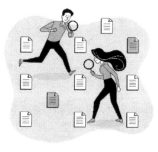

Additionally, many practice tests have a section explaining the answer choices. It can be tempting to read the explanation and think that you now have a good understanding of the concept. However, an explanation likely only covers part of the question's broader context. Even if the explanation makes perfect sense, **go back and investigate** every concept related to the question until you're positive you have a thorough understanding.

As you go along, keep in mind that the practice test is just that: practice. Memorizing these questions and answers will not be very helpful on the actual test because it is unlikely to have any of the same exact questions. If you only know the right answers to the sample questions, you won't be prepared for the real thing. **Study the concepts** until you understand them fully, and then you'll be able to answer any question that shows up on the test.

It's important to wait on the practice tests until you're ready. If you take a test on your first day of study, you may be overwhelmed by the amount of material covered and how much you need to learn. Work up to it gradually.

On test day, you'll need to be prepared for answering questions, managing your time, and using the test-taking strategies you've learned. It's a lot to balance, like a mental marathon that will have a big impact on your future. Like training for a marathon, you'll need to start slowly and work your way up. When test day arrives, you'll be ready.

Start with the strategies you've read in the first two Secret Keys—plan your course and study in the way that works best for you. If you have time, consider using multiple study resources to get different approaches to the same concepts. It can be helpful to see difficult concepts from more than one angle. Then find a good source for practice tests. Many times, the test website will suggest potential study resources or provide sample tests.

Practice Test Strategy

If you're able to find at least three practice tests, we recommend this strategy:

UNTIMED AND OPEN-BOOK PRACTICE

Take the first test with no time constraints and with your notes and study guide handy. Take your time and focus on applying the strategies you've learned.

TIMED AND OPEN-BOOK PRACTICE

Take the second practice test open-book as well, but set a timer and practice pacing yourself to finish in time.

TIMED AND CLOSED-BOOK PRACTICE

Take any other practice tests as if it were test day. Set a timer and put away your study materials. Sit at a table or desk in a quiet room, imagine yourself at the testing center, and answer questions as quickly and accurately as possible.

Keep repeating timed and closed-book tests on a regular basis until you run out of practice tests or it's time for the actual test. Your mind will be ready for the schedule and stress of test day, and you'll be able to focus on recalling the material you've learned.

Secret Key 4: Pace Yourself

Once you're fully prepared for the material on the test, your biggest challenge on test day will be managing your time. Just knowing that the clock is ticking can make you panic even if you have plenty of time left. Work on pacing yourself so you can build confidence against the time constraints of the exam. Pacing is a difficult skill to master, especially in a high-pressure environment, so **practice is vital**.

Set time expectations for your pace based on how much time is available. For example, if a section has 60 questions and the time limit is 30 minutes, you know you have to average 30 seconds or less per question in order to answer them all. Although 30 seconds is the hard limit, set 25 seconds per question as your goal, so you reserve extra time to spend on harder questions. When you budget extra time for the harder questions, you no longer have any reason to stress when those questions take longer to answer.

Don't let this time expectation distract you from working through the test at a calm, steady pace, but keep it in mind so you don't spend too much time on any one question. Recognize that taking extra time on one question you don't understand may keep you from answering two that you do understand later in the test. If your time limit for a question is up and you're still not sure of the answer, mark it and move on, and come back to it later if the time and the test format allow. If the testing format doesn't allow you to return to earlier questions, just make an educated guess; then put it out of your mind and move on.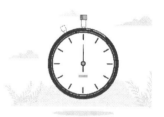

On the easier questions, be careful not to rush. It may seem wise to hurry through them so you have more time for the challenging ones, but it's not worth missing one if you know the concept and just didn't take the time to read the question fully. Work efficiently but make sure you understand the question and have looked at all of the answer choices, since more than one may seem right at first.

Even if you're paying attention to the time, you may find yourself a little behind at some point. You should speed up to get back on track, but do so wisely. Don't panic; just take a few seconds less on each question until you're caught up. Don't guess without thinking, but do look through the answer choices and eliminate any you know are wrong. If you can get down to two choices, it is often worthwhile to guess from those. Once you've chosen an answer, move on and don't dwell on any that you skipped or had to hurry through. If a question was taking too long, chances are it was one of the harder ones, so you weren't as likely to get it right anyway.

On the other hand, if you find yourself getting ahead of schedule, it may be beneficial to slow down a little. The more quickly you work, the more likely you are to make a careless mistake that will affect your score. You've budgeted time for each question, so don't be afraid to spend that time. Practice an efficient but careful pace to get the most out of the time you have.

Secret Key 5: Have a Plan for Guessing

When you're taking the test, you may find yourself stuck on a question. Some of the answer choices seem better than others, but you don't see the one answer choice that is obviously correct. What do you do?

The scenario described above is very common, yet most test takers have not effectively prepared for it. Developing and practicing a plan for guessing may be one of the single most effective uses of your time as you get ready for the exam.

In developing your plan for guessing, there are three questions to address:

- When should you start the guessing process?
- How should you narrow down the choices?
- Which answer should you choose?

When to Start the Guessing Process

Unless your plan for guessing is to select C every time (which, despite its merits, is not what we recommend), you need to leave yourself enough time to apply your answer elimination strategies. Since you have a limited amount of time for each question, that means that if you're going to give yourself the best shot at guessing correctly, you have to decide quickly whether or not you will guess.

Of course, the best-case scenario is that you don't have to guess at all, so first, see if you can answer the question based on your knowledge of the subject and basic reasoning skills. Focus on the key words in the question and try to jog your memory of related topics. Give yourself a chance to bring the knowledge to mind, but once you realize that you don't have (or you can't access) the knowledge you need to answer the question, it's time to start the guessing process.

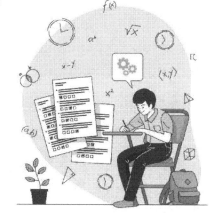

It's almost always better to start the guessing process too early than too late. It only takes a few seconds to remember something and answer the question from knowledge. Carefully eliminating wrong answer choices takes longer. Plus, going through the process of eliminating answer choices can actually help jog your memory.

Summary: Start the guessing process as soon as you decide that you can't answer the question based on your knowledge.

How to Narrow Down the Choices

The next chapter in this book (**Test-Taking Strategies**) includes a wide range of strategies for how to approach questions and how to look for answer choices to eliminate. You will definitely want to read those carefully, practice them, and figure out which ones work best for you. Here though, we're going to address a mindset rather than a particular strategy.

Your odds of guessing an answer correctly depend on how many options you are choosing from.

Number of options left	5	4	3	2	1
Odds of guessing correctly	20%	25%	33%	50%	100%

You can see from this chart just how valuable it is to be able to eliminate incorrect answers and make an educated guess, but there are two things that many test takers do that cause them to miss out on the benefits of guessing:

- Accidentally eliminating the correct answer
- Selecting an answer based on an impression

We'll look at the first one here, and the second one in the next section.

To avoid accidentally eliminating the correct answer, we recommend a thought exercise called **the $5 challenge**. In this challenge, you only eliminate an answer choice from contention if you are willing to bet $5 on it being wrong. Why $5? Five dollars is a small but not insignificant amount of money. It's an amount you could

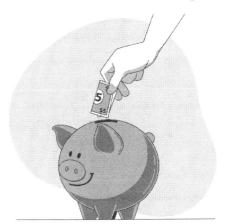

afford to lose but wouldn't want to throw away. And while losing $5 once might not hurt too much, doing it twenty times will set you back $100. In the same way, each small decision you make—eliminating a choice here, guessing on a question there—won't by itself impact your score very much, but when you put them all together, they can make a big difference. By holding each answer choice elimination decision to a higher standard, you can reduce the risk of accidentally eliminating the correct answer.

The $5 challenge can also be applied in a positive sense: If you are willing to bet $5 that an answer choice *is* correct, go ahead and mark it as correct.

Summary: Only eliminate an answer choice if you are willing to bet $5 that it is wrong.

Which Answer to Choose

You're taking the test. You've run into a hard question and decided you'll have to guess. You've eliminated all the answer choices you're willing to bet $5 on. Now you have to pick an answer. Why do we even need to talk about this? Why can't you just pick whichever one you feel like when the time comes?

The answer to these questions is that if you don't come into the test with a plan, you'll rely on your impression to select an answer choice, and if you do that, you risk falling into a trap. The test writers know that everyone who takes their test will be guessing on some of the questions, so they intentionally write wrong answer choices to seem plausible. You still have to pick an answer though, and if the wrong answer choices are designed to look right, how can you ever be sure that you're not falling for their trap? The best solution we've found to this dilemma is to take the decision out of your hands entirely. Here is the process we recommend:

Once you've eliminated any choices that you are confident (willing to bet $5) are wrong, select the first remaining choice as your answer.

Whether you choose to select the first remaining choice, the second, or the last, the important thing is that you use some preselected standard. Using this approach guarantees that you will not be enticed into selecting an answer choice that looks right, because you are not basing your decision on how the answer choices look.

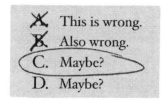

This is not meant to make you question your knowledge. Instead, it is to help you recognize the difference between your knowledge and your impressions. There's a huge difference between thinking an answer is right because of what you know, and thinking an answer is right because it looks or sounds like it should be right.

Summary: To ensure that your selection is appropriately random, make a predetermined selection from among all answer choices you have not eliminated.

Test-Taking Strategies

This section contains a list of test-taking strategies that you may find helpful as you work through the test. By taking what you know and applying logical thought, you can maximize your chances of answering any question correctly!

It is very important to realize that every question is different and every person is different: no single strategy will work on every question, and no single strategy will work for every person. That's why we've included all of them here, so you can try them out and determine which ones work best for different types of questions and which ones work best for you.

Question Strategies

⌀ READ CAREFULLY

Read the question and the answer choices carefully. Don't miss the question because you misread the terms. You have plenty of time to read each question thoroughly and make sure you understand what is being asked. Yet a happy medium must be attained, so don't waste too much time. You must read carefully and efficiently.

⌀ CONTEXTUAL CLUES

Look for contextual clues. If the question includes a word you are not familiar with, look at the immediate context for some indication of what the word might mean. Contextual clues can often give you all the information you need to decipher the meaning of an unfamiliar word. Even if you can't determine the meaning, you may be able to narrow down the possibilities enough to make a solid guess at the answer to the question.

⌀ PREFIXES

If you're having trouble with a word in the question or answer choices, try dissecting it. Take advantage of every clue that the word might include. Prefixes and suffixes can be a huge help. Usually, they allow you to determine a basic meaning. *Pre-* means before, *post-* means after, *pro-* is positive, *de-* is negative. From prefixes and suffixes, you can get an idea of the general meaning of the word and try to put it into context.

⌀ HEDGE WORDS

Watch out for critical hedge words, such as *likely, may, can, sometimes, often, almost, mostly, usually, generally, rarely,* and *sometimes*. Question writers insert these hedge phrases to cover every possibility. Often an answer choice will be wrong simply because it leaves no room for exception. Be on guard for answer choices that have definitive words such as *exactly* and *always*.

13

⊘ Switchback Words

Stay alert for *switchbacks*. These are the words and phrases frequently used to alert you to shifts in thought. The most common switchback words are *but, although,* and *however*. Others include *nevertheless, on the other hand, even though, while, in spite of, despite,* and *regardless of*. Switchback words are important to catch because they can change the direction of the question or an answer choice.

⊘ Face Value

When in doubt, use common sense. Accept the situation in the problem at face value. Don't read too much into it. These problems will not require you to make wild assumptions. If you have to go beyond creativity and warp time or space in order to have an answer choice fit the question, then you should move on and consider the other answer choices. These are normal problems rooted in reality. The applicable relationship or explanation may not be readily apparent, but it is there for you to figure out. Use your common sense to interpret anything that isn't clear.

Answer Choice Strategies

⊘ Answer Selection

The most thorough way to pick an answer choice is to identify and eliminate wrong answers until only one is left, then confirm it is the correct answer. Sometimes an answer choice may immediately seem right, but be careful. The test writers will usually put more than one reasonable answer choice on each question, so take a second to read all of them and make sure that the other choices are not equally obvious. As long as you have time left, it is better to read every answer choice than to pick the first one that looks right without checking the others.

⊘ Answer Choice Families

An answer choice family consists of two (in rare cases, three) answer choices that are very similar in construction and cannot all be true at the same time. If you see two answer choices that are direct opposites or parallels, one of them is usually the correct answer. For instance, if one answer choice says that quantity x increases and another either says that quantity x decreases (opposite) or says that quantity y increases (parallel), then those answer choices would fall into the same family. An answer choice that doesn't match the construction of the answer choice family is more likely to be incorrect. Most questions will not have answer choice families, but when they do appear, you should be prepared to recognize them.

⊘ Eliminate Answers

Eliminate answer choices as soon as you realize they are wrong, but make sure you consider all possibilities. If you are eliminating answer choices and realize that the last one you are left with is also wrong, don't panic. Start over and consider each choice again. There may be something you missed the first time that you will realize on the second pass.

⊘ Avoid Fact Traps

Don't be distracted by an answer choice that is factually true but doesn't answer the question. You are looking for the choice that answers the question. Stay focused on what the question is asking for so you don't accidentally pick an answer that is true but incorrect. Always go back to the question and make sure the answer choice you've selected actually answers the question and is not merely a true statement.

⊘ Extreme Statements

In general, you should avoid answers that put forth extreme actions as standard practice or proclaim controversial ideas as established fact. An answer choice that states the "process should be used in certain situations, if…" is much more likely to be correct than one that states the "process should be discontinued completely." The first is a calm rational statement and doesn't even make a definitive, uncompromising stance, using a hedge word *if* to provide wiggle room, whereas the second choice is far more extreme.

⊘ Benchmark

As you read through the answer choices and you come across one that seems to answer the question well, mentally select that answer choice. This is not your final answer, but it's the one that will help you evaluate the other answer choices. The one that you selected is your benchmark or standard for judging each of the other answer choices. Every other answer choice must be compared to your benchmark. That choice is correct until proven otherwise by another answer choice beating it. If you find a better answer, then that one becomes your new benchmark. Once you've decided that no other choice answers the question as well as your benchmark, you have your final answer.

⊘ Predict the Answer

Before you even start looking at the answer choices, it is often best to try to predict the answer. When you come up with the answer on your own, it is easier to avoid distractions and traps because you will know exactly what to look for. The right answer choice is unlikely to be word-for-word what you came up with, but it should be a close match. Even if you are confident that you have the right answer, you should still take the time to read each option before moving on.

General Strategies

⊘ Tough Questions

If you are stumped on a problem or it appears too hard or too difficult, don't waste time. Move on! Remember though, if you can quickly check for obviously incorrect answer choices, your chances of guessing correctly are greatly improved. Before you completely give up, at least try to knock out a couple of possible answers. Eliminate what you can and then guess at the remaining answer choices before moving on.

⊘ CHECK YOUR WORK

Since you will probably not know every term listed and the answer to every question, it is important that you get credit for the ones that you do know. Don't miss any questions through careless mistakes. If at all possible, try to take a second to look back over your answer selection and make sure you've selected the correct answer choice and haven't made a costly careless mistake (such as marking an answer choice that you didn't mean to mark). This quick double check should more than pay for itself in caught mistakes for the time it costs.

⊘ PACE YOURSELF

It's easy to be overwhelmed when you're looking at a page full of questions; your mind is confused and full of random thoughts, and the clock is ticking down faster than you would like. Calm down and maintain the pace that you have set for yourself. Especially as you get down to the last few minutes of the test, don't let the small numbers on the clock make you panic. As long as you are on track by monitoring your pace, you are guaranteed to have time for each question.

⊘ DON'T RUSH

It is very easy to make errors when you are in a hurry. Maintaining a fast pace in answering questions is pointless if it makes you miss questions that you would have gotten right otherwise. Test writers like to include distracting information and wrong answers that seem right. Taking a little extra time to avoid careless mistakes can make all the difference in your test score. Find a pace that allows you to be confident in the answers that you select.

⊘ KEEP MOVING

Panicking will not help you pass the test, so do your best to stay calm and keep moving. Taking deep breaths and going through the answer elimination steps you practiced can help to break through a stress barrier and keep your pace.

Final Notes

The combination of a solid foundation of content knowledge and the confidence that comes from practicing your plan for applying that knowledge is the key to maximizing your performance on test day. As your foundation of content knowledge is built up and strengthened, you'll find that the strategies included in this chapter become more and more effective in helping you quickly sift through the distractions and traps of the test to isolate the correct answer.

Now that you're preparing to move forward into the test content chapters of this book, be sure to keep your goal in mind. As you read, think about how you will be able to apply this information on the test. If you've already seen sample questions for the test and you have an idea of the question format and style, try to come up with questions of your own that you can answer based on what you're reading. This will give you valuable practice applying your knowledge in the same ways you can expect to on test day.

Good luck and good studying!

18

Cardiovascular Anatomy and Physiology

THE HUMAN HEART

The heart is located in the chest cavity between the lungs. It is located behind the sternum and anterior mediastinum, above the diaphragm, and in front of the vertebral column, esophagus, and posterior mediastinum. The heart sits approximately one to two centimeters left of the midline of the body. The left lung is slightly smaller than the right lung since the heart protrudes into the left side of the chest cavity. The apex of the heart is at the fifth intercostal space at the left midclavicular line. The superior vena cava, inferior vena cava, pulmonary artery, pulmonary vein, and aorta lie above the heart. The aortic arch is situated behind the heart.

Simply, the human heart may be described as a pear-shaped muscle that is about the size of an adult fist. In normal adults, the heart is approximately 12 centimeters in length, eight to nine centimeters in width, and six centimeters thick. The total weight is approximately 250 to 350 grams, depending on age and gender. The weight and size of the heart increases through life into advanced age. The increase in size is more pronounced in men than women.

> **Review Video: BEST Mnemonics for Heart Anatomy and Physiology**
> Visit mometrix.com/academy and enter code: 849489
>
> **Review Video: How the Heart Functions | Anatomy and Physiology Review**
> Visit mometrix.com/academy and enter code: 569724

THE PERICARDIUM

The pericardium is a double-layered sac that contains the heart. The outermost layer is the fibrous pericardium. This dense layer is made of fibrous, connective tissue and acts to protect the heart, anchor it to surrounding walls, limit its movement, and prevent the heart from overfilling with increased blood volume. The fibrous pericardium is continuous with the outer adventitial layer of the vena cava, the aorta, and the pulmonary artery. The innermost layer, or serous pericardium, is thinner and more fragile than the fibrous pericardium and is made of two layers. Both layers of the serous pericardium are composed of a single layer of flat cells. Both the outer or parietal layer and the inner or visceral layer act to lubricate the heart, decreasing friction and absorbing shock during the heart's activity. The pericardial cavity is the space between the parietal and visceral layers and contains serous or pericardial fluid.

19

THE EPICARDIUM

The innermost layer of the pericardium, or visceral pericardium, is also known as the epicardium. It is a cone-shaped sac that envelops the heart. The epicardium is a thin, flat layer of cells consisting of connective tissue covered by fat. It covers the outer surface of the myocardium and forms a protective cover for the heart. In addition to producing pericardial fluid to act as a lubricant and shock absorber for the heart, the epicardium contains the vessels that supply blood to the myocardium.

During ventricular contraction, the wave of depolarization moves from the endocardium to the epicardium.

THE MYOCARDIUM

The myocardium is the middle, muscular layer of the heart. The myocardium is surrounded on the outside by the epicardium and lined on the inside by the endocardium. It is composed of cardiac muscle. Cardiac muscle is also termed "striated," since it appears to be striped when viewed under a microscope. Cardiac muscle is involuntary and requires no input from the central nervous system to contract. In addition to its ability to contract, the myocardium is also able to conduct electrical impulses. The myocardium acts to stimulate the heart to pump blood from the ventricles to the body, and relaxes the atria to allow for the collection of blood.

THE ENDOCARDIUM

The endocardium lines the myocardium and is the innermost layer of the heart. It is a thin, smooth membrane composed of a layer of endothelial cells. It forms a continuous lining that covers the inner surfaces of the heart and heart valves. The endocardium is continuous with the inner lining of large blood vessels. The endocardium also contains Purkinje fibers that participate in the contraction of heart muscle in the myocardium. Purkinje fibers are modified cardiac cells that rapidly conduct electrical signals to the apex of the heart. This ensures that ventricular contraction starts from the base of the heart and spreads up the walls of the ventricles. During the ventricular contraction, a wave of depolarization moves from the inner endocardium to the outer epicardium of the heart.

RIGHT ATRIUM

The atria are thin-walled muscular structures that receive blood returning to the heart. The atria, in turn, pump blood to the ventricles. The right atrium receives blood from the body via the superior and inferior vena cava. The inferior vena cava carries blood from the lower torso and legs to the heart, while the superior vena cava carries blood from the head and upper body to the heart. The right atrium receives blood that is carrying no oxygen. The right atrium is the larger of the two atria and receives a larger volume of blood than the left atrium. The right atrium is capable of expanding in order to accommodate the large volume of blood it receives while maintaining low pressure (0-3 mmHg). The right atrium is separated from the right ventricle by the tricuspid valve.

RIGHT VENTRICLE

The ventricles receive blood from the atria, and then pump blood out of the heart at high pressure. The ventricles have thick, rigid, muscular walls compared to the atria. The right ventricle receives blood from the right atrium as the atrium contracts and pushes blood through the tricuspid valve. When the right ventricle is full of blood the ventricle contracts. The tricuspid valve closes, to prevent blood from flowing back into the atrium, and the pulmonary valve opens, to allow blood to enter the pulmonary artery. The blood flows to the lungs through the pulmonary artery to receive oxygen. The ventricles are not capable of expanding to accommodate large volumes like the atria. The ventricles maintain high pressure in order to forcefully expel blood out of the heart. The right ventricle pumps a smaller amount of blood than the left ventricle and, therefore, is composed of walls that are not as thick as the walls of the left ventricle.

LEFT ATRIUM

The atria are thin-walled muscular structures that receive blood returning to the heart. The atria, in turn, pump blood to the ventricles. The left atrium receives oxygen-carrying blood from the lungs via four pulmonary veins: right inferior, right superior, left inferior, and left superior. The left atrium is capable of expanding to accommodate large volumes of blood, but not to the extent of the right atrium. The left atrium expands to maintain low pressure while receiving large volumes, but maintains higher pressure than the right atrium (6-10 mmHg compared to 0-3 mmHg). The left atrium is separated from the left ventricle by the mitral, or bicuspid, valve.

LEFT VENTRICLE

The ventricles receive blood from the atria, and then pump blood out of the heart at high pressure. The ventricles have thick, rigid, muscular walls compared to the atria. The left ventricle receives blood from the left atrium as the atria contracts and pushes blood through the mitral or bicuspid valve. When the left ventricle is full of blood the ventricle contracts. The mitral valve closes, to prevent blood from flowing back into the atrium, and the aortic valve opens, to allow blood to enter the aorta. The oxygen-carrying blood flows to the entire body by way of the aorta.

The ventricles are not capable of expanding to accommodate large volumes like the atria. The ventricles maintain high pressure in order to forcefully expel blood out of the heart. The left ventricle pumps a larger amount of blood than the right ventricle and, therefore, is composed of thick, muscular walls capable of generating high pressure.

CARDIAC VALVES

The heart contains four valves: two atrioventricular valves and two semilunar valves. The atrioventricular (AV) valves separate the atria from the ventricles. The tricuspid valve separates the right atrium and right ventricle; the mitral, or bicuspid, valve separates the left atrium and left ventricle. The AV valves are flap-like structures made of endocardium and connective tissue that control blood flow within the heart, allowing it to move in only one direction. AV valves have fibrous strands called chordae tendineae that attach the valve to the muscles in the ventricle walls that contract during ventricular contraction. The fibrous strands generate tension and prevent the valve from bulging back into the atrium.

The semilunar valves separate the ventricles from the large blood vessels leading away from the heart. The pulmonary valve separates the right ventricle from the pulmonary artery; the aortic valve separates the left ventricle from the aorta. The semilunar valves are made of three crescent-shaped, or half-moon-shaped, flaps of endocardium and connective tissue.

Semilunar valves differ from atrioventricular valves in that the semilunar valves have no tension-building fibers similar to the chordae tendineae to prevent expansion or bursting of the valves. Semilunar valves ensure unidirectional blood flow out of the heart and are similar to the valves found in veins.

CONTROL MECHANISMS FOR CARDIAC OUTPUT

The cardiac output is determined by multiplying the heart rate (number of beats per minute) and the stroke volume (volume of blood pumped with each heartbeat.) Changes in heart rate or stroke volume, therefore, affect the cardiac output. The stroke volume is controlled by both intrinsic and extrinsic factors. Intrinsic factors include the heart's ability to change its output, or stroke volume, in response to its input. Extrinsic factors include contractility, the strength of cardiac contractions. The contractility is independent of the volume in the ventricle. Heart rate is determined by spontaneous depolarization of the sinoatrial (SA) node. Depolarization at the SA node can be controlled by outside influences, including hormones, electrolytes, body temperature, and the autonomic nervous system.

CARDIAC BLOOD FLOW

The chambers and valves of the heart operate to ensure that blood flows in one direction through the heart and always follows the same path. First, the heart receives blood. Oxygen-poor blood flows from the body into the right atrium through the inferior and superior vena cava. Next, the blood flows from the right atrium into the right ventricle. Next, blood is pumped from the right ventricle to the lungs through the pulmonary artery to receive oxygen from the lungs. From the lungs, the blood flows back to the heart via the pulmonary veins. The left atrium receives this oxygen-rich blood. The blood is then pumped from the left ventricle and through the aorta to the rest of the body.

> **Review Video: Heart Blood Flow**
> Visit mometrix.com/academy and enter code: 783139

HEART SOUNDS

Four distinct heart sounds can be heard throughout the cardiac cycle when recorded with a sensitive phonocardiogram. Typically, only two heart sounds can be heard with a stethoscope.

The first heart sound, S1, is the closing of the atrioventricular valves and signals the beginning of systole. The second heart, S2, sound is the closing of the semilunar valves and marks the end of systole. The third and fourth heart sounds cannot always be discerned with an ordinary stethoscope. The third heart sound, S3, is commonly heard in children and the young adults, or in patients with heart failure. It is the sound of the ventricle filling shortly after S2. Finally, the fourth heart sound, or S4, is caused by the atrium contracting just before S1. It can be heard in patients with weak ventricles.

Important Terms

Ischemia is defined as the lack of oxygen delivery to an organ due to the obstruction or constriction of blood vessels. In myocardial ischemia, the left ventricle does not receive enough oxygenated blood. Atherosclerosis is a common cause of myocardial ischemia. The fatty plaque deposited in the coronary arteries in atherosclerosis causes an obstruction to adequate blood flow. If ischemia persists and the hearts continues to receive an inadequate blood supply, injury or infarction can occur in the heart muscle.

Myocardial injury occurs after a prolonged period of myocardial ischemia. If the heart muscle cannot recover adequate oxygen supply, injury and death to the myocardial tissue can occur. Myocardial injury and ischemia are both reversible processes, if diagnosed early in its progression. Myocardial infarction is the death of myocardial cells causes permanent damage to the heart muscle. The damaged portion of the heart is no longer able to conduct electrical impulses.

Myocardial infarction is commonly known as a heart attack, and may lead to sudden death.

Peripheral resistance: the measure of the total resistance in all the arterioles; changes in peripheral resistance can alter blood pressure

Baroreceptors/Chemoreceptors: receptors in the aortic arch and carotid sinus that sense changes in blood pressure; baroreceptors increase sympathetic tone to decrease heart rate, contractility, and dilation of blood vessels in order to lower blood pressure; baroreceptors decrease the stimulation of the sympathetic nervous system in the presence of low blood pressure.

Anterior or **Ventral**: near or on the front of the body

Posterior or **Dorsal**: near or on the back of the body

Superficial: toward the surface of the body

Peripheral: toward the periphery of the body; located away from the center of the body

External: located on the outside of the body

Internal: located on the inside of the body

Distal: located away from the center of the body

Proximal: located nearest to the center of the body

Superior: toward the head or toward the surface of the body; synonymous with "cephalic"

Inferior: toward the feet or tail or away from the surface of the body; synonymous with "caudal"

Medial: middle or near the middle of the body

Lateral: to the side of the body

Visceral: the covering of the surface of the body or an organ

Parietal: the wall of the surface of the body or organ

Sagittal: lengthwise plane that divides the body into left and right sections

Transverse or **horizontal**: crosswise cut that runs parallel to the ground and divides the body into upper and lower sections

Compliance: the measure of the ability of a vessel to expand and accommodate large volumes

Preload: the amount of tension in a muscle while at rest; in heart muscle, it is determined by end-diastolic volume

Afterload: the amount of tension in a muscle after it begins to contract; in heart muscle, it is determined by aortic pressure

Contractility: the strength of cardiac contractions; independent of the volume in the ventricle; an extrinsic control mechanism for cardiac output

Systemic Circulation

Systemic circulation is the system of blood vessels that carries blood from the heart to all parts of the body, except the lungs. After the heart receives oxygen-carrying blood from the lungs, it pumps the blood out of the heart, first into the aorta, the large blood vessel leading away from the heart. As the arteries move away from the heart, they branch and become smaller vessels: large arteries, small arteries, and arterioles. They continue to deliver oxygen to the body and branch to even smaller vessels, capillaries. The capillaries are the sites of oxygen exchange. The blood vessels then get larger and larger, become venules, then veins. The venous system returns blood to the heart that has delivered its oxygen to the body. The veins deliver oxygen-poor blood to the heart to be pumped to the lungs to receive oxygen again.

> **Review Video: Functions of the Circulatory System**
> Visit mometrix.com/academy and enter code: 376581

ARTERIES AND ARTERIOLES

As the arteries move away from the heart carrying oxygen-rich blood, they branch and become smaller vessels: large arteries, small arteries, and arterioles. The large arteries are 1.0 to 4.0 millimeters in diameter and function to distribute blood through the systemic circulatory system. When the large artery reaches the organ to which it supplies blood, it branches into smaller vessels. The small arteries branch from the large arteries and are 0.5 to 1.0 millimeter in diameter and also function in the distribution of blood, but also generate resistance in the circulatory system to regulate blood pressure and flow rate.

Arterioles branch from the small arteries and are 0.01 to 0.50 millimeters in diameter. They function to regulate resistance in the circulatory system. The arteries are composed of smooth muscle, but as the vessels become smaller, they lose much of the smooth muscle.

MAJOR SYSTEMIC ARTERIES

Systemic circulation is the system of blood vessels that carries blood from the heart to all parts of the body, except the lungs. After the heart receives oxygen-carrying blood from the lungs, it pumps the blood out of the heart, first into the aorta, the large blood vessel leading away from the heart. First, the coronary arteries branch from the root of the aorta and deliver oxygenated blood to the heart muscle. Three other major arteries stem from the aortic arch and supply blood to the head and upper body: carotid and subclavian arteries. Several other major arteries stem from the aorta: renal arteries to supply blood to the kidneys, the celiac and superior and inferior mesenteric arteries to supply the intestines, spleen, and liver, and the iliac arteries, to supply the lower body. The iliac arteries branch to become the femoral and popliteal arteries of the legs.

MAJOR CORONARY ARTERIES

Coronary arteries branch from the root of the aorta and supply the heart muscle with oxygen. There are two coronary arteries, with the left main artery being larger than the right coronary artery. The left main coronary artery divides into two main branches, the left anterior descending artery and the left circumflex artery. The left anterior descending artery supplies the front of the heart, the bottom of the left ventricle, with oxygen-rich blood, while the left circumflex artery wraps around the left side of the heart and supplies the side and back of the left ventricle with blood. The right coronary artery also supplies the back of the heart, namely the right atrium, right ventricle, and part of the left ventricle. Blockage of the coronary arteries leads to heart attacks, heart failure, chest pain, and sudden death.

VENULES AND VEINS

Once oxygen and nutrients are delivered to the body through the capillaries, the blood must be returned to the heart to be pumped to the lungs to receive more oxygen. The small capillaries join together to form venules, which, in turn, join together to form veins to deliver blood to the heart. The venules are approximately 0.01 to 0.50 millimeters in diameter, and function to collect blood and expand and contract to maintain appropriate blood flow in a body region. The venules join together to form veins that are 0.5 to 5.0 millimeters in diameter. The veins also function to regulate the proper flow of blood. Finally, the veins join to the vena cava, which carries blood to the right atrium of the heart. The smallest blood vessels are composed almost entirely of endothelial tissue, but as the venules and veins increase in size, the smooth muscle composition increases.

MAJOR SYSTEMIC VEINS

Systemic circulation is the system of blood vessels that carries blood from the heart to all parts of the body, except the lungs. After the blood has traveled through the body and delivered its oxygen, it must return to the heart to be pumped to the lungs to exchange carbon dioxide for oxygen. Veins are the blood vessels that return blood from the body to the heart. The inferior vena cava returns blood from the legs and torso. The superior vena cava, composed of the subclavian veins, from the arms, and the jugular veins, from the head and neck, return blood to the heart from the upper body. The iliac veins return blood from the legs, hepatic veins from the liver, and renal veins from the kidneys.

MAJOR CORONARY VEINS

Coronary veins return blood to the heart chambers after it has delivered oxygen to the heart muscle through coronary arteries. The coronary venous system is composed of the right and left cardiac venous systems. The left cardiac venous system is composed of several veins: great cardiac vein, middle cardiac vein, small cardiac vein, left marginal vein, left posterior ventricular vein, and the oblique vein. The right cardiac venous system is composed of anterior cardiac veins and right marginal vein. All of the coronary veins deliver blood directly into the right atrium through the coronary sinus, a valve in the right atrium covered by a small flap. The coronary veins run parallel to the coronary arteries on the surface of the heart.

CAPILLARIES

Capillaries are small blood vessels that branch from the arterioles in the systemic circulatory system. While arteries and arterioles are composed, in part, of smooth muscle, capillaries are composed of entirely endothelial cells. They are the smallest vessels within the circulatory system and function as the exchange site for oxygen in the body. In addition, exchange of carbon dioxide, water, electrolytes, proteins, and metabolic waste products are takes place in the capillaries. Capillaries are 0.006 to 0.01 millimeters in diameter. The capillaries join to form venules and veins that deliver the oxygen-poor blood back to the heart.

Blood Pressure

MEAN ARTERIAL PRESSURE

Mean arterial pressure (or MAP) is calculated by adding one-third of the pulse pressure to the diastolic pressure:

$$\text{MAP} = \frac{1}{3}(\text{pulse pressure}) + (\text{diastolic pressure})$$

The MAP may also be calculated by adding the systolic pressure to twice the diastolic pressure and dividing by three:

$$\text{MAP} = \frac{(2 \times \text{diastolic}) + (\text{systolic})}{3}$$

This calculation is not an average of the systolic and diastolic blood pressures, but generates an estimate of the geometric mean blood pressure. In the second equation, diastolic pressure accounts for twice as much as systolic pressure since the heart spends approximately two-thirds of the cardiac cycle in diastole and one-third in systole. An MAP of 60 mmHg is needed to maintain proper blood flow to the major organ systems. The usual range for MAP is 70-110 mmHg.

PULSE PRESSURE

Pulse pressure is the difference between systolic blood pressure and diastolic blood pressure. Diastolic blood pressure is the minimum pressure reached in the arterial system, when blood flows out of the arteries. Systolic blood pressure is the maximum pressure reached, when the ventricle contracts. The pulse pressure is regulated by stroke volume and the elasticity of the arteries. Therefore, the pulse pressure indicates the force of contraction of the ventricles as well as the flexibility of the artery walls. Any change in pulse pressure is likely due to a change in the force of ventricle contraction; the elasticity of the arteries is fairly constant. A change in artery elasticity over a period of years is usually indicative of heart disease.

MEASURING BLOOD PRESSURE

A blood pressure measurement is the amount of force applied to the walls of the arteries during the cardiac cycle. The auscultatory method using a

27

sphygmomanometer is the most common way to measure blood pressure. In this scenario, a patient should be seated with both feet on the floor. The arm is bent slightly and may be supported by a table or armrest. The cuff of the sphygmomanometer is wrapped around the upper arm, with the bottom of the cuff approximately one inch above the elbow, and inflated to approximately 200 mmHg. The pressure created by the cuff temporarily collapses the brachial artery and stops blood flow through it. A stethoscope is placed over the brachial artery in the elbow as the cuff is slowly deflated by two to three mmHg per second. As the pressure in the cuff decreases to the systolic pressure in the artery, a sound is heard that corresponds to the rush of blood through the artery. This pressure when the first sound is heard is recorded as the systolic pressure. As the pressure in the cuff continues to fall, blood continues to flow through the artery. When the pressure in the cuff falls below the diastolic pressure, no more sounds are heard. The pressure when the last sound is heard is recorded as the diastolic pressure.

PRESSURE DIFFERENCES IN THE HEART

In order for blood to flow from the atria to the ventricles, there must be a pressure difference between the atria and the ventricles, since blood flows from higher-pressure environments to lower pressure ones. The left ventricle maintains the highest pressure, followed by the left atrium. Next follows the pressure in the right ventricle, followed by the right atrium. The left ventricle must maintain the highest pressure in order to pump blood to the entire body. The left atrium expands to maintain low pressure (6-10 mmHg) while receiving large volumes, but not to the extent of the right ventricle. The right ventricle is able to maintain lower pressure since it is only pumping blood to the lungs. The right atrium is capable of expanding in order to accommodate the large volume of blood it receives while maintaining low pressure (0-3 mmHg).

AORTIC PULSE PRESSURE

The pressure of the aorta at its highest point, as blood flows out of the left ventricle into the aorta, is, on average, 120 mmHg. The pressure slowly decreases as the ventricle stops pumping blood through the aorta, the semilunar valve closes, and the left ventricle relaxes. The difference between the highest pressure (systolic pressure) and lowest pressure (diastolic pressure) in the aorta is termed aortic pulse pressure.

The aortic pulse pressure is influenced by, first, the ability of the aorta to expand to accommodate the large volume of blood being forced into it by the left ventricle and, second, the volume of blood pumped with each ventricle contraction. For example, an aorta that is very flexible will have a smaller pulse pressure for a given stroke volume than an aorta that is more rigid. A larger stroke volume will result in a larger pulse pressure, regardless of the flexibility of the vessel. Further, the flexibility of the aorta decreases with age, leading to a gradual increase in aortic pulse pressure.

CONTROL MECHANISMS FOR STROKE VOLUME

The cardiac output is determined by multiplying the heart rate (number of beats per minute) and the stroke volume (volume of blood pumped with each heartbeat.) Changes in heart rate or stroke volume, therefore, affect the cardiac output. The stroke volume is controlled by both intrinsic and extrinsic factors. Intrinsic factors include the heart's ability to change its output, or stroke volume, in response to its input. The Frank-Starling Law defines this phenomenon and asserts that, simply, the heart will pump whatever volume of blood it receives. Extrinsic factors include contractility, the strength of cardiac contractions. The contractility is independent of the volume in the ventricle. Most factors affecting contractility affect the level of calcium inside the cell. These factors include drugs or the autonomic nervous system.

DETERMINING CARDIAC OUTPUT

Cardiac output is the amount of blood pumped from the left ventricle through the aorta to the rest of the body in one minute. Since the right and left sides of the heart must pump the same amount of blood over a given period of time, the average output of the right ventricle is equal to that of the left ventricle. The average cardiac output for a resting adult male is 5 liters per minute. The stroke volume is the amount of blood pumped with each heartbeat. This can be calculated by finding the difference between the end-diastolic volume and the end-systolic volume. The cardiac output is, therefore, found by multiplying the stroke volume by the number of beats per minute: $CO = HR \times SV$.

Electrical Conduction System

The electrical conduction system of the heart generates and propagates the electrical impulses that sustain the rhythmic electrical contractions of the heart. The entire system is composed of the sinoatrial (SA) and atrioventricular (AV) nodes and the internodal pathways, the Bundle of His, as well as the right and left bundle branches and the anterior and posterior fascicles. First, the SA node generates a spontaneous electrical impulse that stimulates atrial contraction, corresponding to the P wave on the ECG. Next, the electrical impulse reaches the AV node and slows in velocity. This corresponds to the PR segment on the ECG. The electrical impulse travels through the Bundle of His and the bundle branches, then to the Purkinje fibers. The Purkinje fibers carry the electrical impulse that stimulate the ventricles to depolarize and contract, corresponding to the QRS complex.

> **Review Video: Electrical Conduction System of the Heart**
> Visit mometrix.com/academy and enter code: 624557

CONTROL MECHANISMS FOR HEART RATE

The cardiac output is determined by multiplying the heart rate (number of beats per minute) and the stroke volume (volume of blood pumped with each heartbeat.) Changes in heart rate or stroke volume, therefore, affect the cardiac output. Heart rate is determined by spontaneous depolarization of the sinoatrial (SA) node. Depolarization at the SA node can be controlled by outside influences, including hormones, electrolytes, body temperature, and the autonomic nervous system. For example, norepinephrine and acetylcholine are transmitters within the autonomic nervous system and act to increase or decrease the heart, respectively. Increasing the heart rate results in limited effects on cardiac output. First, the upper limit of heart rate is approximately 250 beats per minute. Second, with rapid heart rates, cardiac output actually decreases. There is not enough time in between beats for the ventricles to fill with blood, so each beat pumps less blood to the body.

SINOATRIAL NODE

The electrical conduction system of the heart generates and propagates the electrical impulses that sustain the rhythmic contractions of the heart. The entire system is composed of the sinoatrial (SA) and atrioventricular (AV) nodes and the internodal pathways, the Bundle of His, as well as the right and left bundle branches and the anterior and posterior fascicles. The SA node is often called the "pacemaker" of the heart. The SA node is the site of the spontaneous generation of the electrical impulse that stimulates the heart to contract. The SA node is an oblong-shaped group of muscle cells in the right atrium. It is the larger of the two nodes acting in the electrical conduction pathway. The SA node typically generates a heartbeat at a rate of 60 to 100 beats per minute, but can be influenced by the autonomic nervous system to increase or decrease the heart rate.

MEASUREMENT SITES OF HEART RATE AND BLOOD PRESSURE

Typically, blood pressure is measured using the auscultatory method. A sphygmomanometer is used, with the cuff placed above the elbow on the upper arm and inflated. A stethoscope is placed over the brachial artery to listen for sounds as the pressure changes as the cuff is deflated. A normal systolic blood pressure is 120 mmHg, while a normal diastolic is 80 mmHg. The heart rate may be measured at any place on the body where an artery is close to the surface. For example, the heart rate may be measured at the radial artery in the wrist, the carotid artery in the neck, the brachial artery in the elbow, or the femoral artery in the groin. A normal heart rate ranges from 60 to 100 beats per minute.

INTERNODAL PATHWAY

The electrical conduction system of the heart generates and propagates the electrical impulses that sustain the rhythmic contractions of the heart. The entire system is composed of the sinoatrial (SA) and atrioventricular (AV) nodes and the internodal pathways, the Bundle of His, as well as the right and left bundle branches and the anterior and posterior fascicles.

The internodal pathway carries electrical impulses from the SA node to the AV node. The internodal pathway also carries the electrical impulse to both the right and left atria and stimulates atrial contraction. This conduction occurs rapidly because the muscle cells of the atria are large and have a large negative resting potential. This produces a very rapid depolarization and subsequent conduction of electrical impulse.

ATRIOVENTRICULAR NODE

The electrical conduction system of the heart generates and propagates the electrical impulses that sustain the rhythmic contractions of the heart. The entire system is composed of the sinoatrial (SA) and atrioventricular (AV) nodes and the internodal pathways, the Bundle of His, as well as the right and left bundle branches and the anterior and posterior fascicles. The AV node is located in the lower portion of the right atrium. The AV node receives the electrical impulse generated by the SA node via the internodal pathway. As the electrical potential arrives at the AV node, it slows in velocity and is delayed at the AV node for approximately 0.1 seconds before traveling to the Bundle of His. The delay is required to ensure that the atria have completed their contraction before the ventricles begin contracting.

RIGHT AND LEFT BUNDLE BRANCHES

The electrical conduction system of the heart generates and propagates the electrical impulses that sustain the rhythmic contractions of the heart. The entire system is composed of the sinoatrial (SA) and atrioventricular (AV) nodes and the internodal pathways, the Bundle of His, as well as the right and left bundle branches and the anterior and posterior fascicles. The Bundle of His divides to form the right and left bundle branches. The right bundle branch carries electrical impulses to the right ventricle and the left bundle branch carries electrical impulses to the left ventricle. Electrical conduction through the bundle branches is very rapid.

BUNDLE OF HIS

The electrical conduction system of the heart generates and propagates the electrical impulses that sustain the rhythmic contractions of the heart. The entire system is composed of the sinoatrial (SA) and atrioventricular (AV) nodes and the internodal pathways, the Bundle of His, as well as the right and left bundle branches and the anterior and posterior fascicles. After the electrical impulse is slowed in the AV node, the impulse passes to the Bundle of His. The Bundle is composed of thin, specialized muscle cells that connect the distal portion of the AV node to the right and left bundle branches. The Bundle of His is specialized for very rapid electrical conduction and the electrical impulse travels at its highest speed through the Bundle.

PURKINJE FIBERS

The electrical conduction system of the heart generates and propagates the electrical impulses that sustain the rhythmic contractions of the heart. The entire system is composed of the sinoatrial (SA) and atrioventricular (AV) nodes and the internodal pathways, the Bundle of His, as well as the right and left bundle branches and the anterior and posterior fascicles.

The bundle branches divide into the Purkinje fibers, located in the walls of both the right and left ventricles. These fibers form a network over the surface of the heart and penetrate into the muscles of the ventricles. The Purkinje fibers deliver the electrical impulse that stimulates ventricular depolarization and contraction. The Purkinje fibers maintain a high velocity of electrical conduction.

ANTERIOR AND POSTERIOR FASCICLES

The electrical conduction system of the heart generates and propagates the electrical impulses that sustain the rhythmic contractions of the heart. The entire system is composed of the sinoatrial (SA) and atrioventricular (AV) nodes and the internodal pathways, the Bundle of His, as well as the right and left bundle branches and the anterior and posterior fascicles. The left bundle branch is very short and almost immediately divides into the anterior and posterior fascicles. The posterior fascicle carries the electrical impulse to the inferior and posterior portions of the left ventricle. The anterior fascicle carries electrical impulses to the anterior and superior portions of the left ventricle. The posterior fascicle is short and broad, in relation to the anterior fascicle, and it particularly resistant to ischemic damage.

HEART RATE FACTORS

The sinoatrial (SA) node is often called the "pacemaker" of the heart. The SA node is the site of the spontaneous generation of the electrical impulse that stimulates the heart to contract. The SA node typically generates a heartbeat at a rate of 60 to 100 beats per minute, but can be influenced by the autonomic nervous system to increase or decrease the heart rate.

Substances from the sympathetic nervous system, norepinephrine (noradrenaline) and epinephrine (adrenaline) may stimulate the SA node. In this case, the depolarization of the SA node occurs more quickly, and more action potentials are generated, leading to an increased heart rate. If the SA node is stimulated by acetylcholine, the rate of depolarization is decreased, leading to a decreased heart rate.

Conducting Preprocedural Activities

Verifying the Physician's Orders

PROTOCOL FOR VERIFYING THE PHYSICIAN'S ORDERS FOR STRESS TESTING

The technician should review the patient's chart ahead of the scheduled stress test. Ideally, this should be done at least one day prior to the test. The chart should be reviewed to ensure that the physician has indeed ordered the stress test and to confirm the diagnosis for which it is being performed, which type of stress test has been ordered, and that the patient is reasonably expected to be able to tolerate the test. The chart should be assessed for prior medical issues such as arthritis or lung disease, which may prevent the patient from achieving the target heart rate during the test. The patient should be contacted to discuss the test; should be briefed on what to expect before, during, and after the test; and should be allowed to ask questions about the test. Additionally, the patient should be instructed about whether to eat or drink prior to the test and about which medications should not be taken in advance of the test. However, physician preferences may vary, and the technician should become familiar with the protocol of the usual ordering physicians.

ASSESSING PATIENT LIMITATIONS

Prior to beginning an exercise stress test, the technician should assess the patient's ability to complete the test safely. Medical conditions that may prevent completion of exercise stress testing include severe arthritis, extremity amputation, severe peripheral vascular disease, chronic obstructive pulmonary disease, and general debility. In the presence of any of these conditions, the ordering physician should consider switching the patient to a pharmacologic stress test.

Contraindications to pharmacologic stress testing include asthma with ongoing wheezing or bronchospasm, second- or third-degree heart block without the presence of a pacemaker, systolic blood pressure <90 mmHg, and caffeine use within 12 hours prior to the test.

Verifying Patient Identifiers

PROPER IDENTIFICATION OF A PATIENT

The proper identification of a patient is vital and should be verified at the start of any clinical encounter. The Joint Commission, a nonprofit organization that accredits US healthcare organizations and programs, established procedures to help ensure the accuracy of patient identification in the clinical setting.

Accordingly, each patient should be identified by at least two of the following:

- Full legal name
- Date of birth
- Medical identification number

This task should be performed immediately upon first encountering the patient, before any procedure is performed.

Patients may have identical names, but their different birthdates and medical identification numbers help to uniquely identify the correct patient.

HIPAA AND ENCOUNTERED ISSUES

The Health Insurance Portability and Accountability Act of 1996 (HIPAA) is a federal law that restricts access to an individual's private medical information. It also limits disclosure of a patient's protected health information. Protected health information includes any electronic, written, or oral clinical data and identifying demographic information including the patient's phone number and social security number. A healthcare worker can use and disclose protected health information for the purpose of treatment, payment, or other healthcare operations. However, only the minimum amount of information should be disclosed to protect the patient's privacy. There are criminal and monetary penalties that can be issued if a healthcare entity is found to be in violation of HIPAA rules.

Obtaining Patient Consent

IMPLIED VS. INFORMED CONSENT

Implied consent is an informal agreement that allows disclosure of health information. An example of this is when a patient schedules an appointment with a physician, he or she gives implied consent for treatment. In contrast, **informed consent** is formal permission obtained from a patient to perform a specific test or procedure. It is voluntary consent obtained prior to any procedure, with the form written in a language understood by the patient that the patient signs and dates.

A **healthcare proxy** is a patient-appointed agent listed in a legal document to serve as a patient's healthcare decision maker if the patient becomes incapable of making his or her wishes known. In many cases, this proxy is a spouse or a parent. A healthcare proxy can be appointed for anyone older than 18 years old. The proxy goes into effect when a physician determines that the patient is incapable of making his or her own medical decisions.

Applying Universal and/or Isolation Precautions

UNIVERSAL PRECAUTIONS

Universal precautions are a set of infectious disease protection guidelines introduced by the Centers for Disease Control in the 1980s, following the AIDS epidemic. Under these guidelines, each patient is assumed to be potentially infected with a bloodborne pathogen. The healthcare worker should take precautions to prevent the spread of infection between patients and to protect himself or herself from contact with potential pathogens as well. This is accomplished with the use of personal protective equipment such as disposable gloves and protective barriers such as goggles and face shields. Additionally, used needles and scalpels should be handled carefully and disposed of in puncture-resistant containers. Frequent handwashing and washing of skin areas that had contact with the patient's bodily fluids are also vital in reducing the risk of pathogen spread.

ISOLATION PRECAUTIONS

Isolation precautions are procedures enacted to separate a sick patient with a contagious disease from healthy people, thus preventing the spread of infection in the general population. This is accomplished by the use of personal protective equipment such as gloves, gowns, and masks worn by the healthcare worker. Additionally, engineering controls can be instituted, such as the use of mechanical or structural barriers to prevent direct contact between an infected patient and a healthcare worker. The use of negative air pressure in hospital rooms can help to control the flow of airborne pathogens.

Performing Patient Transfer and Transport

SAFE PATIENT TRANSFER AND TRANSPORT METHODS

When a patient with a debility or mobility issue presents for stress testing, the technician should allow the patient to assist in his or her own transfer from one location to another as much as possible. The technician's feet should be shoulder width apart, the floor should be free of obstacles, and the patient should be positioned as close to the technician as possible. These efforts help reduce the risk of injury to the technician and to the patient. Additionally, the technician should lift the patient using the legs, not the back, and should avoid twisting the back; instead, he or she should pivot on his or her feet as necessary. The technician's back should be kept straight when lifting because this helps to minimize back strain.

ERGONOMICS

Ergonomics is the science of arranging an efficient and safe work environment. The goal of ergonomics is to reduce the risk of injury to the technician. This is accomplished by putting a number of safeguards into action. A common source of injury to the healthcare worker occurs is heavy lifting of the patient or equipment. The object being lifted should be placed as close to the body as possible to minimize twisting or muscle sprain. The use of mechanical-assist devices and adjustable-height tables also help reduce risk of injury. Additionally, high task repetition should be avoided if possible. Frequent repetitive motion can strain or sprain muscles. The technician should take breaks from repetitive maneuvers as needed and enlist the help of another staff member if needed. Proper ergonomic procedures will help minimize work-related injury to the technician.

USE AND MAINTENANCE OF EQUIPMENT FOR STRESS TESTING

The exercise stress test machine is an expensive and frequently used piece of equipment. It should be cleaned after each patient encounter. Additionally, it should be checked for proper calibration of the blood pressure and heart rate measurements on a regular basis. The treadmill should undergo routine maintenance for optimum functioning. The patient should be briefed prior to the stress test about proper use of the equipment for safety but also to prevent any damage to the machine.

The patient is attached to the electrocardiogram (ECG) electrodes in a supine position, and then he or she is guided to the stationary treadmill and advised to hold on to the railing. The treadmill is started per the Bruce protocol, which begins at a slow pace and with no incline to allow a three-minute warmup period. After adequate exercise, there is a cool-down period in which the speed and incline gradually return to baseline, so the patient does not have to stop exercising abruptly. The patient is then guided back to the exam table, and the ECG electrodes are removed.

Identifying Proper Anatomical Landmarks

ANATOMIC LANDMARKS USED IN PERFORMANCE OF THE 12-LEAD ECG

The standard 12-lead ECG uses 10 electrodes. The four limb leads are

- RA – right arm, anywhere between the right shoulder and right elbow
- LA – left arm – anywhere between the left shoulder and left elbow
- RL – right leg – anywhere between the right torso and above the right ankle
- LL – left leg – anywhere between the left torso and above the left ankle

The limb leads should be placed symmetrically on the right and left sides.

The chest leads are labeled V1–V6, and their anatomic positions are as follows:

- V1 – fourth intercostal space at the right sternal border
- V2 – fourth intercostal space at the left sternal border
- V3 – between V2 and V4
- V4 – fifth intercostal space at the midclavicular line
- V5 – horizontal to V4 at the anterior axillary line
- V6 – horizontal to V4 and V5 at midaxillary line

The angle of Louis, or the sternal notch, is located at the level of the second intercostal space and can be used as a landmark.

Preparing the Patient

PROPER POSITIONING FOR AN ECG

Proper patient positioning is vital to obtaining a high-quality ECG. Informed consent should be obtained prior to the start of the test. Infection-control protocols should be followed, with proper handwashing being performed before touching the patient. The patient should remove any electronic devices from his or clothes because they can produce artifacts on the ECG. The chest and all four limbs should be exposed to ensure proper electrode application. In women, breast tissue can impact the ECG amplitude due to the distance between the electrode and the heart, so lead V4 may need to be placed under the breast. The patient should lie in the semi-recumbent position, with arms flat at the sides, legs uncrossed, and he or she should be instructed to lie still and quiet during the acquisition of data. The patient's privacy should be maintained as much as possible, minimizing exposure of the chest with a blanket or sheet as needed. The electrodes should be removed after completion of the tracing.

PROPER SKIN PREPARATION FOR CARDIAC PROCEDURES

Skin can be a source of artifact for ECG tracings, unless it is properly prepped. The goal is to reduce the skin impedance, thereby reducing the resistance to alternating current electrical signals and producing a clear ECG tracing. The ECG electrode skin site should be cleaned with soap and water, and the area should be dried with a dry cloth. Avoid cleaning the skin with alcohol because this can dehydrate the skin and impede electrical flow. Light exfoliation of the skin site helps remove dead skin cells in the stratum corneum layer of the epidermis, which has high impedance; this allows for better signal transmission. If the patient's chest is very hairy, it may be necessary to clip the hair off to ensure adequate skin contact with the electrode. Additionally, if the patient is wearing lotion on the chest, it should be washed off completely prior to the placement of electrodes.

Equipment Calibration, Maintenance, and Cleaning

CALIBRATION OF MEDICAL EQUIPMENT

Calibration of medical equipment ensures that the output quality is accurate and on par with industry standards. If the machinery is not properly calibrated, this can result in an incorrect diagnosis. Calibration should be performed as recommended by the device manufacturer. Additionally, predetermined calibration intervals should be established, such as monthly or quarterly. Finally, an emergency calibration session should occur if the device has been dropped or damaged. Calibration should be performed by a trained person, either from in house or by a third party. Some facilities have regulations about the calibration of medical devices, requiring documentation and record keeping. Noncompliance with these regulations may result in a fine being assessed.

MAINTENANCE AND CLEANING OF MEDICAL EQUIPMENT

Proper maintenance of medical equipment is important for adequate patient care and from a financial standpoint. Broken equipment increases patients' wait times, can result in canceled appointments, and prevents the facility from providing full patient care. Routine maintenance is vital to ensure that frequently used, expensive medical equipment is functioning at full capacity. In some cases, a financial penalty may result from improper documentation of equipment maintenance. The surfaces of many medical devices can be cleaned with disinfecting wipes. Environmental Protection Agency-approved disposable products with a contact time of one to three minutes are ideal; the device is considered fully disinfected three minutes after cleaning, and it is ready for use on the next patient. Consult the specific medical device's user guide to ensure that these wipes are compatible for use.

CALIBRATION OF THE ECG MACHINE

The standard ECG is calibrated at 10 mm height and recorded at 25 mm/sec. If the machine is set to a different calibration, this can affect the interpretation of the tracing. The baseline ECG should be assessed to ensure that the recording is steady and the printing is clear.

The ECG machine should be dusted daily with a dry cloth, and a dust cover should be placed over it at the end of the day. The ECG machine should be plugged into a power source. The battery, battery indicator, power indicator, and cable connector indicator should be checked for functionality and integrity. The exterior rollers and paper guides should be cleaned and checked daily.

The ECG machine is an expensive piece of machinery that should be handled with care. Avoid pulling or twisting on the wires and cables. The machine should be kept out of heat or direct sunlight; moisture should be avoided. The ECG machine can be put into test mode, which performs a check of the machine and monitor to ensure proper functioning. Finally, the machine should be fully calibrated and serviced by a biomedical technician every six months to ensure its integrity.

CALIBRATION OF THE DEFIBRILLATOR

The defibrillator is a vital piece of equipment whose location should be in close proximity to any stress test room. Its proper functioning must be ensured in case it is required in an emergency. Most machines do daily self-checks and display a warning if a problem is noted. Nonetheless, monthly manual checks should be performed to ensure proper functioning. The electrode pads should be changed after each use and at least every two years if left unused. The battery life is typically two to five years depending on the model. All staff should have adequate training and simulation sessions to ensure familiarity with the specific device model.

CALIBRATION OF THE SPHYGMOMANOMETER

Routine calibration of the blood pressure cuff is essential to proper cardiac care of the patient. The cuff should routinely be examined for cleanliness and to ensure that the plastic housings are intact. Check the security of the attachment of the device to the wall mount (if applicable). Check the line cord, and examine the power cord for damage. Examine the strain relief at both ends of the cord. Check for security of the cables, and ensure that there is no insulation break. Examine the control switches for proper alignment, and ensure that all functions are adequately performing. Check all indicators to ensure proper operation of visual displays. Finally, verify the calibration of the displays.

CLEANING OF THE SPHYGMOMANOMETER

The blood pressure cuff is a medical tool used multiple times daily in a busy clinic. The cuff and tubing are in frequent contact with patients' skin, and they can become soiled with stains, body fluids, and bacteria. To clean the cuff, put on gloves and examine the entire cuff, looking for stains. Remove the tubing from the cuff. Refer to the owner's manual to ensure that the cuff can be soaked in warm, soapy water. Do not soak the tubing. The tubing can be cleaned with antimicrobial disinfecting wipes; the cuff may also be cleaned this way.

MAINTENANCE AND CLEANING PROCEDURE OF THE TREADMILL

The treadmill should be set up on level ground for optimal use. Plug the power cord into an outlet with a surge protector. The treadmill surfaces should be wiped down with a sanitizing cloth after each use. Make sure to clean under the treadmill once per week to prevent accumulation of dust and dirt. Tighten the treadmill belt as needed to maintain tension; refer to the owner's guide for the location of the tightening bolts. Some treadmills have self-lubricating belts; others require intermittent application of a lubricant that is machine-specific. The belt may also need to be realigned periodically, if it appears to be slipping or sliding, by adjusting the bolts located on the back of the machine.

CLEANING OF THE HOLTER MONITOR AND THE ECG MACHINE

The exterior plastic surfaces of the Holter monitor device can be cleaned easily and effectively with bleach wipes or Environmental Protection Agency-approved disposable disinfecting wipes. Do not use bleach on any metal electrical contacts or cables because this can shorten their useful lifespan, and avoid alcohol because this can be drying. Avoid excessive moisture, which can infiltrate and damage the battery or the recording apparatus, and dry the equipment completely before the next use. Refer to the owner's manual of your specific equipment for optimal results.

The ECG machine is used multiple times per day and should be kept clean to minimize the spread of infection. Unless the ECG has single-use wires and clips, the clips should be washed routinely with soap and water and then dried completely. Consult the owner's manual for machine-specific recommendations.

Safety Hazards/Considerations

ENVIRONMENT FOR PERFORMING AN ECG

The ECG is a very common and safe test that provides various types of cardiac information to the ordering physician. The test should be performed in a quiet, private room because the test requires electrodes to be placed on the bare skin of the chest. Although male patients are usually bare-chested for the test, female patients can be given a gown while the electrodes are applied to the chest.

Even though it is rare, a patient may experience redness or itching at the site of the electrode placement due to an allergic reaction to the adhesive on the electrode. This reaction is usually self-limited and resolves on its own.

Performing an ECG

Troubleshooting While Performing the ECG Procedure

TROUBLESHOOTING LEAD REVERSALS OF AN ECG

Lead reversals are very common and affect the quality and accuracy of the ECG. Most commonly, the left- and right-arm leads can be reversed, causing a negative (downward) QRS complex in lead I with a negative P wave in lead I; this is a common cause of right-axis deviation on an ECG. Sometimes, the arm and foot electrodes are switched, leading to a very small QRS complex in lead II or III. Finally, reversal of the chest leads can cause inappropriate R-wave progression, in which the amplitude fluctuates from high to low and back to high.

TROUBLESHOOTING ARTIFACTS ON AN ECG

Artifact is a common ECG problem. This is can be due to muscle movement, twitching, or tremors in Parkinson's patients. The electrode should be adjusted away from a large muscle mass if possible. Additionally, electrical interference from power cords, ventilators, or high impedance from skin can affect the ECG quality. The ECG machine should be moved away from electrical devices if possible. Hair on the skin or dead skin cells cause high skin impedance, which decreases the magnitude of the ECG signal. In an adult, the skin may need to be shaved and it may need to be mechanically abraded to remove dead skin cells on the chest surface prior to placement of the electrode patch in order to ensure an adequate connection.

TROUBLESHOOTING AN INTERMITTENT TRACING ON AN ECG

If a continuous ECG tracing is not being produced, check that the cables are properly placed into the monitor, that the lead wires are properly inserted into the cable, and that the lead wires are well attached to the electrodes. Also, ensure that the electrodes are not old, that the conducting gel has not dried out, and that the skin surfaces have been properly prepared with shaving and abrading as necessary to ensure a good connection to the lead wires. Finally, check for damaged lead wires and replace as needed.

Standard 12-Lead ECG

INFORMATION OBTAINED FROM THE STANDARD 12-LEAD ECG

The 12-lead ECG provides a painless, low-risk, simple, and cost-effective 10-second snapshot of the heartbeat. It provides vital information about the rhythm of the upper and lower chambers of the heart. Additionally, the ECG can tell whether the atria and ventricles are abnormally thickened or enlarged. It can be used to diagnose an active or recent heart attack, show delays in the signaling of the heartbeat from one chamber to another, and provide information about active

40

cardiac inflammation or infection. Finally, it can help diagnose electrolyte abnormalities or other medical conditions such as pulmonary embolism.

Review Video: <u>12 Lead ECG</u>
Visit mometrix.com/academy and enter code: 962539

STEPS IN PERFORMING AN ECG

Prior to performing an ECG, it is imperative to verify the patient's name and birthdate and to ensure that this information is entered correctly on the ECG machine. An ECG uses 10 electrodes that contain conducting gel. Electrodes are attached to the patient's right and left arms and right and left legs, and 6 electrodes are attached across the patient's thorax in the fourth and fifth intercostal spaces from the right of the sternum to the midaxillary line. These areas should be cleaned with alcohol before attaching the electrodes. Hairy areas of the chest may need to be shaved and cleaned to ensure that the electrodes will stick properly to the skin. The electrodes are attached by wires to the ECG machine, information is obtained about the signaling of the heart, and then the information is translated into waveforms on the ECG, which can then be interpreted by the physician. The patient's torso should be covered with a sheet while obtaining the ECG. The technician should review the ECG for the quality of the data, ensuring that there is not excessive motion or a missing recording from one of the leads before disconnecting the electrodes.

EXPECTATIONS OF PATIENTS UNDERGOING AN ECG

A patient undergoing an ECG should be reassured that it is a safe, noninvasive, and quick way to obtain cardiac information. He or she should be advised that the test will provide a myriad of diagnostic information and that the results will be quickly available to the ordering physician.

After confirming the patient's name and birthdate, instruct him or her to remove the clothing from the waist up, as well as any jewelry, watches, and electronic devices that could interfere with the signaling during the ECG. After the electrodes are attached, the patient should be instructed to lay as still as possible and avoid extra movement while the ECG is being obtained. Upon completion of the ECG, the electrodes should be removed, the skin should be wiped off, and the patient should be instructed to get dressed.

Modified ECG

DEXTROCARDIA

Dextrocardia is a rare condition in which the heart is located on the right side of the thorax rather than on the left. The cardiac anatomy is a mirror image of normal. The incidence of this condition is approximately 1 in 12,000 people. In some cases, there is dextrocardia with situs inversus, wherein the heart and the abdominal organs are located in a mirror image of their normal positions.

Because, in dextrocardia, the heart is located on the mirror side of its normal position, the ECG electrodes should be placed on the mirror image of the normal orientation. The left-arm electrode should be placed on the right arm. Precordial chest leads V3–V6 should be placed on the mirror image location of the usual location on the anterior thorax. The patient should be given routine instructions similar to those for a standard ECG.

POSTERIOR ECG

The posterior ECG should be performed when a posterior myocardial infarction (MI) is suspected. This condition can occur in up to 20% of inferior or lateral wall myocardial infarctions, and it is usually supplied by the left circumflex or dominant right coronary artery. A posterior wall MI can be difficult to detect on a standard 12-lead ECG, so a modified ECG is performed and is labeled "posterior ECG." In this type of ECG, leads V1–V3 remain unchanged; V4–V6 are relabeled as V7–V9; lead cable V6 connects to V9, which is located on the patient's back at the left spinal border, in the same horizontal line as V4–V6; V8 connects to lead cable V5 and is located posteriorly at the midscapular line, in the same horizontal line as V7 and V9; V7 connects to lead cable V4 and is located on the patient's back at the midaxillary line, in the same horizontal line as V4–V6; and V6 has no leads attached, but it serves as a reference point for the horizontal placement of V7–V9.

A posterior wall myocardial infarction is seen as an ST elevation of 0.5 to 1 mm in V8–V9. The presence of this finding complicates the clinical scenario and could change clinical decision making.

The ECG should be immediately labeled as "posterior ECG," and V4–V6 should be relabeled as V7–V9 to avoid confusion with a standard ECG. The patient undergoing a posterior ECG should be given the same instructions as for a standard ECG.

RIGHT-SIDED ECG

A right-sided ECG is used to detect an acute right ventricular myocardial infarction. These infarctions account for up to 50% of acute inferior wall myocardial infarctions, which involve right coronary artery occlusion, and can complicate and change the patient's clinical course and treatment. The right-sided ECG is up to 90% sensitive and is specific for diagnosing a right ventricular myocardial infarction.

The decision to perform a right-sided ECG should be made upon seeing ST elevation in leads II, III, and AVF in the standard 12-lead ECG. ST elevation in V1 can also be seen. A right ventricular myocardial infarction is diagnosed if there is ST elevation of 1 mm in lead V4R.

The patient with an acute inferior or right ventricular infarction may be hypotensive and clinically unstable. Nonetheless, he or she should be given instructions similar to those for a standard ECG.

RIGHT-SIDED VS. STANDARD ECG LABELING AND ELECTRODE PLACEMENT

The ECG should immediately be labeled as "right-sided ECG," and the leads should be relabeled V1R–V6R to avoid confusion with a standard 12-lead ECG. The right-sided ECG is performed with the following changes to the electrode placement:

- V1R – located at the fourth intercostal space at the left sternal border
- V2R – located at the fourth intercostal space at the right sternal border
- V3R – located halfway between V2R and V4R on a diagonal line
- V4R – located at the fifth intercostal space, right midclavicular line
- V5R – located at the right anterior axillary line, in the same horizontal line as V4R and V6R
- V6R – located at the right midaxillary line, in the same horizontal line as V5R and V6R

The arm and leg leads remain the same as in a standard 12-lead ECG.

SIGNAL-AVERAGED ECG

The signal-averaged ECG is a diagnostic test that provides a detailed ECG from multiple tracings taken over 10–20 minutes, as opposed to a routine ECG, which records for only a few seconds. The signal-averaged ECG compiles the average of at least 250 QRS complexes in order to detect subtle changes in electrical activity that are not apparent in the standard 12-lead ECG and may occur only intermittently. This requires the filtering out of extraneous noise in the tracing, most commonly from skeletal muscle. This test could reveal small, microvolt variations in the QRS complex, usually called late potentials, that can predispose the patient to dangerous ventricular tachyarrhythmias. The late potentials represent fragmented depolarization of ventricular myocardium that can serve as the substrate for a dangerous arrhythmia. The signal-averaged ECG can help with risk stratification of the patient with a history of myocardial infarction or coronary artery disease to determine if he or she is at a higher risk for sudden cardiac death.

CARDIOPULMONARY EXERCISE TEST

The cardiopulmonary exercise test helps assess the patient's cardiovascular and ventilatory response to exercise. The patient exercises on a stationary bicycle, usually for fewer than 12 minutes, until exhaustion. He or she may be required to breathe through a tube, similar to a pulmonary function test. The blood pressure, pulse oximetry, and ECG tracing are monitored during the test. The information obtained includes blood gas, blood pressure, and oxygen consumption data that help assess the patient's cardiac and pulmonary status.

DOUBLE PRODUCT

The **double product** (also called the rate pressure product) measures the energy demand of the heart during exercise. It helps gauge the intensity of the body's hemodynamic response to exercise. The double product is calculated with the following equation:

[heart rate] × [systolic blood pressure] = double product.

Double Product	Hemodynamic Response
>30,000	High
25,000–29,999	High intermediate
20,000–24,999	Intermediate
15,000–19,999	Low intermediate
10,000–14,999	Low

COURSE OF BLOOD FLOW THROUGHOUT A CARDIAC CYCLE

Deoxygenated blood returns from the various body organs via the superior and inferior vena cava and into the right atrium. From the right atrium, blood travels through the tricuspid valve into the right ventricle and then across the pulmonary valve to the lungs via the pulmonary artery. In the lungs, the blood is reoxygenated and flows via the pulmonary vein into the left atrium, across the mitral valve, and into the left ventricle. The left ventricle is the main pumping chamber of the heart. During systole, the aortic valve opens and blood is expelled from the left ventricle into the aorta, and it flows to the rest of the body to provide oxygen. Subsequently, this blood becomes deoxygenated, and it again returns to the right atrium via the superior and inferior vena cava.

15-Lead Pediatric ECG

PERFORMING A 15-LEAD PEDIATRIC ECG

The pediatric ECG uses the same anatomic positions as the adult ECG. However, in a newborn or an infant, the right ventricle predominates in the chest due to fetal circulation. To better visualize the right ventricle, the right-sided leads V2R–V4R are added. The pediatric ECG limb lead placement is the same as for an adult. Place the electrodes on the top part of the arm or leg for less muscle interference. For the precordial leads, the placement is as follows:

- V1 – fourth intercostal space, right sternal border
- V2 – fourth intercostal space, left sternal border
- V3 – midway between V2 and V4
- V4 – left midclavicular line between ribs 5 and 6
- V5 – anterior axillary line, the same horizontal plane as V4
- V6 – midaxillary line, the same horizontal plane as V4
- V2R – fourth intercostal space, right sternal border
- V3R – diagonally between V2R and V4R
- V4R – fifth intercostal space, right midclavicular line

Pediatric ECG

The pediatric ECG enables the clinician to obtain information on the child's cardiac functioning. Data obtained include the heart rhythm, left or right bundle branch block (RBBB/LBBB), chamber size, and hypertrophy of the cardiac chambers. Rhythm problems such as sinus arrhythmia, supraventricular tachycardia (SVT), and Wolff–Parkinson–White syndrome have characteristic findings on ECG. Diagnosis of RBBB and LBBB is similar to that of an adult. Due to the thinner chest wall in the pediatric patient compared to the adult, the ECG leads are closer to the heart and the voltages can appear exaggerated. Therefore, if using adult ECG criteria, it would appear that there is right or left ventricular hypertrophy; instead, a different set of criteria is used.

Corrected QT Interval

The QT interval refers to the total time from ventricular depolarization to complete repolarization. Increases in the QT interval can cause syncope, torsades de pointes, and sudden cardiac death. The causes of QT interval prolongation can be congenital or acquired, such as due to certain medications or hypokalemia. Because the QT interval shortens as the heart rate increases, a correcting formula was devised to calculate the corrected QT interval, called the QTc interval. This allows for variations in the heart rate.

Data Obtained from the Pediatric ECG

The pediatric ECG differs from the adult ECG in important ways. A resting heart rate of more than 100 beats per minute (bpm) can be normal for children, whereas in an adult this would be considered tachycardic. Also, because the right ventricle is more prominent than the left ventricle in a child, right-axis deviation of greater than 90 degrees can be seen. Additionally, a juvenile T-wave pattern can be observed, in which there is T-wave inversion in leads V1–V3, whereas in an adult this would raise the concern for ischemia. T waves may also be inverted in the right precordial leads. Sinus arrhythmia is common in children, and one may see a dominant R wave or RSR' pattern in lead V1. Additionally, the PR interval and QRS duration may be shorter and the QTc interval may also increase slightly. An abnormally long QTc interval is considered greater than 450 msec in a male and more than 470 msec in a female. If the R wave of V6 intersects with the baseline of V5, this is considered abnormal. Causes of this condition include aortic stenosis, coarctation of the aorta, and ventricular septal defect. Right ventricular hypertrophy should only be diagnosed in lead V1 if there is an R wave in a child older than six months of age or an upright T wave in V1 in a child after the first week of life.

Instructions for the Pediatric Patient

The child needing an ECG is likely to be anxious and can present challenges to obtaining a quality ECG. If possible, a trusted caregiver should be present to help calm the child. Explain the purpose of the test. Advise the patient that the test is painless, relatively short, and it does not involve any injections. Showing the patient the machine and electrodes in advance may be helpful. The limb leads should be placed on the top part of the arm or leg for less muscle interference. The child

45

should be encouraged to remain still during acquisition of data and should be quietly distracted if possible.

Axis Deviations

NORMAL AXIS ON ECG AND DIAGNOSING RIGHT- AND LEFT-AXIS DEVIATION

The QRS axis on an ECG refers to the net direction of the depolarization of the heart's electrical activity. The normal QRS axis on an ECG is between –30 and +90 degrees. The axis is determined by examining lead I and lead AVF and determining the net direction of the QRS complex. If the net deflection of the QRS in leads I and AVF is positive (upright), then the axis is normal. If the net QRS deflection is negative in lead I and positive in AVF, then right-axis deviation is present. Right-axis deviation is between +90 and +180 degrees. This can occur in RBBB, right ventricular hypertrophy, or dextrocardia. Finally, if the net QRS deflection is positive in lead I but negative in lead AVF, then left-axis deviation is present. Left-axis deviation is between –30 and –90 degrees. This can be seen as a normal variant, left ventricular hypertrophy, or LBBB. Rarely, extreme axis deviation can be seen (also called the northwest axis), which is between –90 and –180 degrees. This can be caused by reversal of the right-arm and left-leg leads or in ventricular tachycardia (VT).

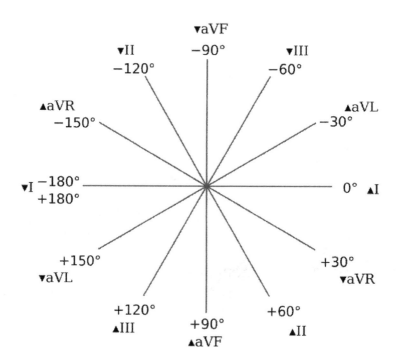

DIAGNOSING RIGHT- AND LEFT-AXIS DEVIATIONS ON AN ECG

Right-axis deviation is present when the QRS axis is between +90 and +180 degrees. The QRS (dominant R wave) is positive in leads II, III, and AVF. Causes of right-axis deviation include a normal pediatric patient, dextrocardia, chronic obstructive pulmonary disease (COPD), pulmonary embolus, RBBB, or right ventricular hypertrophy.

Left-axis deviation on ECG occurs with a QRS axis of less than –30 degrees. The QRS complex is positive (dominant R wave) in lead I and negative (dominant S wave) in leads II, III, and AVF. Common causes of left-axis deviation include LBBB, ventricular pacing, inferior wall myocardial infarction, and left ventricular hypertrophy.

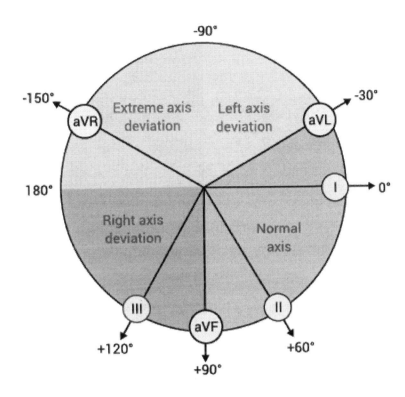

Bundle Branch Blocks (RBBB/LBBB)

PATHOPHYSIOLOGY, ECG MORPHOLOGY, AND COMMON CAUSES OF RIGHT AND LEFT BUNDLE BRANCH BLOCK (RBBB/LBBB)

In the normal heart, the right and left ventricles depolarize simultaneously via the right and left bundle branches. In the presence of either a right or left bundle branch block (RBBB/LBBB), the signal propagates normally through one side of the heart but the depolarization of the other side occurs more slowly, leading to a widening of the QRS morphology on ECG tracings of greater than 0.12 seconds. In an RBBB, the right ventricle is depolarized more slowly than the left ventricle. Common causes of RBBB include cardiomyopathy, right ventricular hypertrophy, and congenital heart disease such as atrial septal defect.

In the presence of an LBBB, the left ventricle is depolarized more slowly than the right ventricle. The presence of an LBBB is always considered pathologic. It can imitate an acute myocardial infarction and can mask ischemia on ECG, due to the presence of ST- and T-wave changes that are similar in myocardial infarction and in LBBB. Common causes of LBBB include left ventricular hypertrophy, congestive heart failure, and hypertension. It is important to determine if the LBBB is chronic, based on prior ECGs if they are available, or if it is a new-onset LBBB. In the setting of chest pain or shortness of breath, the new onset of an LBBB could actually be an acute myocardial infarction.

Hypertrophy

CAUSES AND ECG CRITERIA OF RIGHT AND LEFT VENTRICULAR HYPERTROPHY

Hypertrophy refers to abnormal thickening of the cardiac chamber, due to abnormal pressure overload. This can lead to suboptimal pumping capability, resulting in shortness of breath, chest pain, or arrhythmia. Right ventricular hypertrophy can be caused by lung disease such as pulmonary hypertension, congenital heart diseases such as pulmonic stenosis, or tricuspid regurgitation. The ECG criteria for right ventricular hypertrophy are the following: right-axis deviation of at least 110 degrees, R-wave dominance over the S wave in V1–V2, and S-wave dominance over the R wave in lead V6. Additionally, there are secondary ST-T-wave changes in V1–V2 that are discordant (in the opposite direction) to the QRS complex. Right-atrial enlargement, called P pulmonale, can also be seen.

In contrast, left ventricular hypertrophy is commonly caused by hypertension or aortic valve disease. On ECG tracings, clues to the presence of left ventricular hypertrophy include left-axis deviation and left-atrial enlargement, called P mitrale.

The Sokolow–Lyon criteria for left ventricular hypertrophy are either of the following:

- R-wave amplitude in V5 or V6 plus S-wave amplitude in V1 or V2 greater than 35 mm
- R-wave amplitude in lead aVL greater than 11 mm

There are also secondary ST-T-wave changes in V5, V6, and leads I and aVL, with downsloping ST segments and inverted T waves. The ST segments in leads V1 and V2 are elevated and slightly concave.

ECG Morphology

ANATOMIC LOCATIONS OF THE ECG LEADS AND ARTERIES SUPPLIED BY EACH

The leads of the ECG are grouped according to the coronary artery that they supply. These groupings are called contiguous leads. Leads I and aVL are the lateral limb leads, and they are supplied by the left circumflex artery or the left anterior descending artery. Lead aVL stands for the augmented unipolar left arm lead; it faces the heart from the left side and is oriented to the anterior lateral surface of the left ventricle. Leads II, III, and aVF are the inferior leads, usually supplied by the right coronary artery. Lead aVF stands for the augmented unipolar left leg, and it is oriented to the inferior surface of the heart. Leads V1–V2 are the septal leads, supplied by the left anterior descending artery. Leads V3–V4 are the anterior leads, also supplied by the left anterior descending artery. Finally, leads V5–V6 are the lateral leads, supplied by the left circumflex artery. The ability to localize these leads is vital in the setting of ischemia or infarction because this helps pinpoint the coronary artery being acutely compromised. Lead aVR is the augmented unipolar R arm lead; it faces the heart from the right side and displays reciprocal information to that of leads aVL, II, and V5–V6.

DIFFERENT MORPHOLOGIES OF THE T WAVE AND THEIR SIGNIFICANCE

The T-wave represents ventricular repolarization on the ECG. It should be positive (have an upward deflection) in most leads. The T-wave should be concordant with the preceding QRS, meaning that if the QRS has a net positive deflection, so should the T-wave. T-wave inversion without ST segment depression or elevation does not represent ischemia. However, if there is T-wave inversion in two contiguous leads with ST depression or elevation, this is abnormal and could represent current or recent ischemia. However, T-wave inversion can also be seen in bundle branch block, ventricular pacing, or left ventricular hypertrophy. Large, symmetric, pointy, upright T waves >10 mm in males or >8 mm in females could indicate hyperkalemia.

NORMAL AND ABNORMAL Q WAVES ON ECG AND THEIR SIGNIFICANCE

The Q wave is the first negative deflection preceding the R wave on an ECG. It represents the normal left-to-right depolarization of the interventricular septum. Small Q waves, measuring <1 mm in duration and less than 25% of the R-wave amplitude, can be normal in most ECG leads except in leads V1–V3. Pathologic Q waves are defined as being >1 mm wide, >2 mm deep, or >25% of the QRS depth, or a Q wave seen in leads V1–V3. The pathologic Q wave should be seen in at least two contiguous leads to be considered significant. This indicates current or prior myocardial infarction. The pathologic Q wave can be seen in association with ST elevation or depression or with T-wave inversion indicating an ischemic event. The differential diagnosis for pathologic Q waves includes myocardial infarction; cardiomyopathy including hypertrophic cardiomyopathy; or lead placement error, e.g., an upper limb lead being placed on a lower limb.

Ischemic Changes/Infarction

ISCHEMIC MORPHOLOGY ON THE ECG

In the setting of acute ischemia, when a coronary artery's blood flow is being compromised but not completely occluded, certain ECG changes occur. These usually take the form of horizontal ST-segment depression (at least 0.5 mm of depression using the PR segment as a baseline) and T-wave inversion in contiguous ECG leads; if not quickly reversed, a non-ST-segment elevation myocardial infarction can occur, in which the subendocardial tissue can be permanently damaged, or infarcted. Medications such as beta blockers, nitroglycerin, and clopidogrel can be used to help restore blood flow, but a definitive invasive procedure called angioplasty and cardiac stenting may be necessary.

INFARCTION MORPHOLOGY ON THE ECG

In the case of an ST-segment elevation myocardial infarction, the coronary blockage is complete, encompassing the entire left ventricular wall thickness from endocardium to epicardium. Failure to reverse this situation quickly can cause infarction of the affected heart area, leading to permanent heart weakness. Emergency angioplasty is usually needed. The classic ECG findings of ST-elevation myocardial infarction are the following: ST-segment elevation resembling a "fireman's hat," or a convex-shaped morphology in at least two adjacent ECG leads.

The culprit lesion, meaning the coronary artery that is being blocked and is causing the ischemia, can usually be localized based on the ECG leads that show the ST elevation; for example, ST elevation in leads II, III, and aVL correspond to an inferior wall myocardial infarction caused by occlusion of the right coronary artery.

Performing Stress Tests

Stress Test Supplies and Equipment

SUPPLIES AND EQUIPMENT REQUIRED FOR STRESS TESTING

The technician should have reviewed the patient's chart and verified that the stress test has been ordered and that the correct patient is being evaluated. The treadmill should have been turned on and assessed for proper functioning. The display screen should be evaluated to ensure that the data will be recorded properly. Ensure that there is adequate recording paper on the machine. A manual blood pressure cuff should be used to record the patient's blood pressure, and the tubing should be inspected ahead of the test to ensure that it is functioning normally. Make sure you have a pen to record the blood pressure readings. Confirm that a defibrillator is located nearby in case of emergency.

PERFORMING THE TREADMILL STRESS TEST

The patient should be attached to the electrodes, a resting 12-lead ECG is performed, and baseline blood pressure and heart rate readings are recorded. The treadmill should be started according to the Bruce protocol, which includes a warm-up period. The ECG is constantly displayed on the screen, and it is recorded at 1-minute intervals for later review. The patient should be encouraged to exercise to exhaustion, or at least until obtaining the predetermined target heart rate based on age. He or she should be asked about the perceived level of exertion at each stage, according to the Borg scale, and monitored for any concerning symptoms or ECG abnormalities. Finally, the patient should be monitored for symptoms during the recovery stage, for about five minutes post exercise.

PERFORMING THE BICYCLE STRESS TEST

The bicycle stress test is more commonly performed in Europe. It is a less intense form of exercise test compared to the treadmill stress test. Advantages of bicycle stress testing over treadmill stress testing include lower cost, smaller space requirement for the equipment, less tracing artifact, and ease of hearing and measuring the blood pressure during the test. The resistance of the bicycle is measured in watts (W). The test starts at 40 W for females and 50 W for males. Every other minute, the resistance is increased by 15 W for women and by 15–30 W for men. The total test duration is usually 7–10 minutes. The main drawback of the bicycle test is that it requires strong quadriceps muscles; the exercise tolerance is limited if the patient has pain or weakness in this muscle group.

ERGOMETRY STRESS TEST

The ergometer or arm cycle is an alternative to routine treadmill or bicycle stress testing. It is used in patients with paraplegia or lower extremity disability. The patient can sit or stand while cranking an arm ergometer. The test is graded, with increases in workload occurring every two minutes until exhaustion. Two protocols are available, one more vigorous, one less vigorous, depending on the patient's

51

exercise tolerance. The test can include simultaneous oxygen consumption measurement.

SINGLE-PHOTON EMISSION COMPUTER TOMOGRAPHY IMAGING METHOD

Single-photon emission computer tomography imaging is performed using a gamma camera. The camera captures emitted radiation from injected radioisotopes to create 3D images of the heart. Prior to exercising on the treadmill, the patient is injected with a radioisotope (technetium or thallium) and he or she lies down under the gamma camera for a set of resting cardiac images. At peak exercise on the Bruce protocol, the patient is again injected with another dose of the radioisotope, and another set of images is obtained with the gamma camera. The before-and-after exercise images are compared. If differences are detected in blood flow, this can suggest ischemia. Prior myocardial infarction can also be detected by comparing these images. Further cardiac testing may be ordered for evaluation.

Stress Test Protocol

BRUCE PROTOCOL

The Bruce protocol is a safe, standardized exercise regimen developed by Dr. Robert Bruce in 1963. It is composed of seven stages on a treadmill, each lasting three minutes. These stages are designed to assess the patient's level of exercise fitness and blood pressure and heart rate response to exercise and to unmask coronary ischemia by using a continuous ECG tracing at rest, during exercise, and in the recovery stages.

The standard Bruce protocol regimen is listed below:

Stage	Speed (mph)	Grade (%)	METS (metabolic equivalents)
Rest	0.0	0	1.0
1	1.7	10	4.6
2	2.5	12	7.0
3	3.4	14	10.1
4	4.2	16	12.9
5	5.0	18	15.1
6	5.5	20	16.9
7	6.8	22	19.2

PROCEDURE FOR THE BRUCE PROTOCOL STRESS TEST

After verification of the patient's demographics, the patient's chest should be cleaned and electrodes should be attached, according to the ECG protocol. A resting ECG, resting blood pressure, and heart rate measurements are obtained. The patient is instructed to walk or run on the treadmill until exhaustion, with the goal heart rate being 85% of maximum capacity, which is obtained by the formula

$$[220 - (\text{patient's age})] \times 0.85.$$

The blood pressure and heart rate readings are recorded at each successive stage of exercise. The patient should be monitored closely and asked about his or her perceived level of exertion and any symptoms of chest discomfort, dizziness, or shortness of breath. Monitoring should continue for approximately five minutes after the cessation of exercise.

INSTRUCTIONS FOR AND EXPECTATIONS OF A PATIENT

The patient undergoing a Bruce protocol treadmill stress test should be instructed to wear comfortable clothing and shoes in which he or she will be able to walk or run safely. He or she should be advised to stop medications such as beta blockers, which can prevent the achievement of the target heart rate, according to the protocol of the ordering physician. Cardiac stimulants such as alcohol or caffeine should also be avoided for 12 hours before the test. The patient is instructed to walk or run on the treadmill to exhaustion or until development of symptoms such as chest pain or shortness of breath. He or she may hold onto the treadmill railings lightly. Proper performance of the stress test allows the maximum diagnostic data to be attained.

The patient is expected to follow the preparatory instructions provided by the staff. These include instructions about which medications to stop in advance of the test, the avoidance of cardiac stimulants, and fasting on the morning of the test. Additionally, the patient is expected to exercise to exhaustion, to provide as much data as possible for the ordering physician.

BORG RATING OF PERCEIVED EXERTION SCALE

The Borg Rating of Perceived Exertion scale is a standardized method of determining the patient's subjective estimates of exercise intensity during stress testing, with levels of 6–20. High perceived exertion at a low level of exercise is a strong predictor of adverse outcomes. The patient should be asked to rate his level of exertion at the various stages of exercise.

Exertion Description	Borg Rating
None	6
Very, very light	7 to 8
Very light	9 to 10
Fairly light	11 to 12
Somewhat hard	13 to 14
Hard	15 to 16
Very hard	17 to 18
Very, very hard	19 to 20

MODIFIED BRUCE PROTOCOL

The modified Bruce protocol is an adjusted version of the standard Bruce protocol that is geared toward elderly or sedentary patients who would have a difficult time tolerating the increasing treadmill speed and incline of the Bruce protocol. In contrast to the Bruce protocol, in which the speed of the treadmill increases every three minutes, the modified Bruce protocol speed stays constant at 1.7 mph. Additionally, the incline is less steep, starting at 0% and increasing to 10%. The patient exercises to exhaustion, as in the Bruce protocol, and is monitored with continuous ECG and interval measurement of blood pressure and heart rate. The patient must reach 85% of the age-predicted maximum heart rate in order for the test to be considered diagnostic.

A patient undergoing a modified Bruce protocol stress test should be informed that he or she should exercise to exhaustion, but that the test is designed to be achievable for his or her level of fitness. The patient should wear comfortable clothes and shoes conducive to exercise and should not take beta blockers or drink alcohol for 24 hours prior to the test.

DUKE TREADMILL SCORE (DTS)

The Duke treadmill score (DTS) is a health tool that gives prognostic information about coronary artery disease based on the treadmill stress test. The score on the DTS ranges from –11 to +15, with a lower score predicting a higher risk of coronary artery disease. The DTS is calculated by the following equation:

[exercise time (min)] − [5 × ST deviation (mm)] − [4 × anginal index].

The exercise time is the number of minutes completed on the Bruce protocol.

The ST deviation is the maximum ST depression or elevation in any lead other than aVR, with abnormal being >1 mm of the ST deviation.

The anginal index is based on the following score: 0 for no angina experienced during the test, 1 for nonlimiting angina, and 2 for exercise-limiting angina.

Score Range	Interpretation
Higher than +5	A 97% survival rate at five years and considered low risk for CAD.
Between –11 and +4	Intermediate risk for CAD, with a five-year survival rate of 90%.
Between –25 and –11	High risk for CAD, with a five-year survival rate of 65%.

METABOLIC EQUIVALENT (MET)

The metabolic equivalent (MET) is an estimation of the energy cost of physical activity. One MET is defined as the amount of oxygen consumed while sitting at rest, which is 3.5 mL oxygen per kilogram per minute. The MET describes the patient's functional capacity during stress testing and is associated with the prognosis; the higher the MET level achieved on stress testing, the better the prognosis.

Examples of MET workloads include the following:

Level	MET	Example Activity
Light work	<3	Sitting, washing dishes
Moderate work	3–6	Swimming, brisk walking, yardwork
Vigorous work	>6	Bicycling, playing tennis, running

ABSOLUTE TERMINATION CRITERIA DURING EXERCISE STRESS TESTING

Absolute termination of exercise stress testing should occur with

- A drop in the systolic blood pressure (SBP) greater than 10 mm with other signs of ischemia including chest pain and shortness of breath
- SBP>220 mmHg
- Presence of angina
- Dizziness or presyncope
- Cyanosis or pallor
- The patient's desire to stop
- Technical problems with the ECG machine or BP cuff making recording of data unreliable
- VT >30 seconds
- SVT with hemodynamic changes
- ST elevation of 1 mm or more in a lead without prior Q waves
- ST depression of 2 mm or more in two contiguous leads

NAUGHTON PROTOCOL

The Naughton protocol is a treadmill stress test protocol that is used on sedentary adults who have lower than average exercise tolerance. It is implemented to help diagnose the presence of coronary artery disease.

In contrast to the standard Bruce protocol for routine exercise stress testing, the Naughton protocol has shorter stages (each two minutes long), provides a two-minute warmup, maintains a constant low speed of 2 mph instead of incrementally increasing, and has a less steep incline, increasing by 3.5% per stage. The goal with the Naughton protocol is not to obtain the maximum heart rate, but instead to attain 80–90% of the maximum heart rate.

The patient should be instructed to wear comfortable clothes and shoes for exercising and should not take beta blockers or drink alcohol for 24 hours prior.

Pharmacological / Nuclear Stress Test Protocols

PHARMACOLOGICAL NUCLEAR STRESS TEST

The pharmacologic stress test should be performed to evaluate for coronary artery disease in a patient who is either unable to exercise on a treadmill due to orthopedic issues, has general debility, has a pacemaker, or has certain types of abnormal ECGs including LBBB. Instead of exercising, the patient is injected with a vasodilator, such as adenosine or regadenoson (Lexiscan). These chemicals can unmask areas of decreased cardiac blood flow without the patient having to obtain a certain level of exercise. Before and after the injection of the vasodilator, a radioactive tracer, commonly technetium-99m sestamibi (Cardiolite) or technetium-99m tetrofosmin (Myoview), is injected and a gamma camera obtains images of the heart. When these images are compared, areas of cardiac stenosis can become apparent.

The patient should be instructed to avoid alcohol for 24 hours prior to the test and to avoid caffeine for 12 hours prior to the test. Potential side effects of the vasodilator include dizziness, flushing, and nausea, although these are usually short in duration.

DOBUTAMINE STRESS ECHO

The dobutamine stress echo is a stress test that should be considered to evaluate for coronary artery disease in a patient who has severe COPD or reactive airway disease. Nuclear pharmacologic stress testing with adenosine or regadenoson (Lexiscan) is contraindicated in these patients because it can exacerbate bronchospasm.

Instead, resting echocardiographic images are obtained with the patient lying supine, and then the patient is injected with escalating doses of dobutamine, a beta agonist that increases the heart rate and contractility of the heart, mimicking exercise. A second set of echocardiographic images is obtained when the peak heart rate is achieved. The images are reviewed for areas of regional or global wall motion abnormalities, which can indicate coronary artery disease.

The patient should be instructed to avoid the use of beta blockers for 24 hours prior to the test because this interferes with the dobutamine activity. The patient may feel flushing, palpitations, or dizziness during the test, which all usually resolve after the dobutamine infusion is complete.

EXERCISE NUCLEAR STRESS TEST

The exercise nuclear stress test is performed to determine the presence of coronary artery disease. It is approximately 10–15% more accurate than a regular exercise stress test. It should be considered in a patient with a prior history of coronary artery disease, if the patient is having intermittent episodes of chest discomfort despite a normal regular exercise stress test, or in other clinical cases as determined by the ordering physician.

An intravenous line is inserted, and the patient receives a radiotracer chemical, usually Tc 99 sestamibi. The patient lies on a table, and a gamma camera takes a set of resting cardiac images in various orientations. The patient then exercises on the treadmill while connected to a continuous ECG machine, using the Bruce protocol to achieve the target heart rate based on age. After exercise, a second set of cardiac images is obtained with the gamma camera. The pre- and postexercise images are compared, and abnormalities in cardiac blood flow can be detected with approximately 80–85% accuracy.

The patient should be instructed to avoid beta blocker medication and alcohol for 24 hours prior to the test. He or she should wear comfortable clothes and shoes that are appropriate for exercise.

Performing Ambulatory Monitoring

Ambulatory Monitoring Supplies and Equipment

The physician order for the proper test should be obtained, and the patient's information should be verified. The technician should obtain alcohol pads, a razor, electrodes, the correct type of monitor device, tape, lead wires, cables, and a patient diary to log symptoms. A man's chest hair may need to be shaved in the areas where the electrodes need to be placed to ensure a good seal.

The ambulatory monitoring device, whether a Holter or event monitor, should be checked for battery life, integrity of the cables and wires, and freshness of the electrode gel. Ensure that the cables and electrodes are fully attached and inserted into their proper locations. If any of these parameters are suboptimal, it can affect the data obtained.

Once the patient is attached to the monitoring device, press the event button to cycle through channels 1, 2, and 3 to verify the ECG amplitude and to ensure the good shape and clarity of the signal. The patient should walk in place, and the tracing should be reviewed to ensure that there is no artifact or muscle noise; and if so, new electrodes should be placed. Be sure to check that the patient's name and identification number are written in any patient diary or log.

METHODS OF ATTACHING LEADS FOR AMBULATORY ECG MONITORING

Patients undergoing ambulatory ECG monitoring must have secure attachment of the electrodes; the device will not yield usable data if the leads are detached. Therefore, it is important that the electrodes are applied correctly and securely at the start of the monitoring period. The skin should be prepped and cleaned with alcohol if it is oily to ensure good contact and a good seal of the electrode with the skin. Ensure that there are no wrinkles on the electrode pad; otherwise, remove and replace it. A stress loop is formed by taping a loop of the electrode wire to the patient's chest to pick up the slack of the wire, so it is less likely to get caught on something and detach. There still should be some slack in the wire to allow the patient to move freely without the electrode being pulled off.

A fabric pouch is sometimes used to hold the monitor. It can be worn around the neck or over the shoulder to allow the patient to move more freely during the monitoring period.

REMOVING ECG LEAD ADHESIVE

The residual adhesive from ambulatory ECG leads may be hard to remove. If soap and water do not adequately remove the adhesive, rubbing alcohol should help.

Some patients may report stinging, burning, or soreness at the site of skin contact with the ECG electrode. This may appear as a small bump, or it may look similar to a burn. This is most often a nonallergic irritation due to the chemical in the adhesive, also called contact dermatitis. The treatment is to remove the irritating adhesive completely by gently cleaning with soap and water. Ideally, the skin should be left uncovered, but it can be gently covered with a sterile gauze if needed. The patient should avoid similar adhesives in the future.

While allergic dermatitis is less common, it can have a similar appearance to contact dermatitis as well as itching at the adhesive site. Topical steroids may be prescribed in these cases after evaluation by a physician. If skin blisters develop, a physician should be contacted for further evaluation.

Ambulatory Monitoring Equipment and Procedure Troubleshooting

HOLTER MONITOR

The Holter monitor is an ambulatory ECG monitor used to detect and diagnose heart rhythm abnormalities when they occur. It enables the physician to see what type of heart rhythm is occurring at the time of symptoms, and it helps to guide treatment. This type of monitor is best for patients having symptomatic palpitations or dizziness at least once per day. The Holter monitor is typically worn for 24–48 hours. To set up the Holter monitor, screw the lead wires into the recorder. The patient's name and the recorder's serial number should be written onto the memory card and the patient diary. New batteries should be installed. The leads should be applied. The common five-lead Holter monitor consists of an RA (white) lead, placed near the right midclavicular line, directly below the clavicle. The LA (black) lead is placed near the left midclavicular line, directly below the clavicle. The V1 lead (brown) is placed to the right of the sternum at the fourth intercostal space. The LL (red) lead is placed between the sixth and seventh intercostal spaces on the L midclavicular line. Finally, the RL (green) lead is placed between the sixth and seventh intercostal spaces on the right midclavicular line.

INSTRUCTIONS FOR AND EXPECTATIONS OF PATIENTS

The patient scheduled for a Holter monitor should be advised to wear a loose-fitting shirt. He or she should be advised to record the type of symptoms and the day and time of occurrence onto the patient diary provided. The diary is subsequently compared with abnormal heart rhythms on review of the Holter monitor to check for correlation. The patient should be instructed not to open up the monitor, not to touch the electrodes or lead wires, and to keep all parts of the apparatus dry at all times.

The Holter device should be checked for problems or malfunctions before the patient exits the office. Common problems include artifact or muscle noise, which may require repositioning with new electrodes; intermittent tracing or no tracing, which could be due to dry electrodes; or damaged lead wires or cables, which should be replaced. The technician should also check to ensure that the cable is fully attached to the monitor and that the lead wires are securely attached to the electrodes.

EVENT MONITOR

The event monitor is a type of ambulatory ECG recording device typically used for patients having intermittent, random symptoms of palpitations or dizziness that may not happen on a daily basis. Therefore, a longer length monitor is required to increase the chances of catching the rhythm on paper, which aids in diagnosis and treatment. Commonly, the event monitor is worn for 30 days; however, it can be removed for showering.

When preparing to apply an event monitor to a patient, install new batteries into the monitor. The monitor is placed on the patient using the same anatomic landmarks as used for the Holter monitor. The patient's name, as well as the date, should be recorded on the memory card. The recording device is worn on a belt or a shoulder strap. When a symptomatic episode occurs, the patient presses a button to active the device, which records the ECG tracing for a predetermined time prior to the event, the event itself, and a certain time length after the event (usually up to five minutes). This information is then transmitted to the ordering physician for evaluation.

INSTRUCTIONS FOR PATIENTS

The patient with an event monitor should be shown how to activate the device using the recording button. He or she should be told to keep the device dry and to not open the recorder. The patient can shower after removing the device, and after the shower he or she should reapply it. The patient should be instructed to push the recording button for any episode of palpitations or dizziness to enable the physician to arrive at a diagnosis of the symptoms.

The event monitor should be checked before the patient leaves the office to ensure that there is no artifact or muscle noise on the recording. If there is, this may require repositioning the leads with new electrodes. Ensure that the lead wires are securely attached to the electrodes and that the cables are fully attached to the monitor.

INITIATING A PATIENT ON THE TELEMETRY MONITOR

Telemetry is a type of ambulatory ECG monitoring typically used in an inpatient setting such as a hospital. The patient can be continuously monitored for heart rate and oxygen saturation while being allowed to ambulate short distances around the room or the hospital hallway. The electrode leads are attached to the patient. The skin should be prepped appropriately as needed to ensure a good ECG signal, similar to the procedure for a routine ECG. The patient wears a five-lead device with electrode placement similar to that of the Holter monitor, which includes RA, LA, V1, LL, and RL leads. The electrode lead wires are attached to the telemetry unit. The telemetry device is programmed from the central monitoring center to display information at the bedside. A technician watches the telemetry data in real time, 24 hours per day and notifies the nursing staff if there is a rhythm abnormality reaching predetermined alarm criteria. The monitoring device is usually worn around the neck.

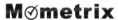

INSTRUCTIONS FOR PATIENTS

The patient being placed on telemetry should be told that the heart rhythm will be continuously monitored. The patient should be instructed not to get the monitoring device wet and not to open the monitor. The patient should stay within the boundary of the telemetry unit while ambulating and should only ambulate under supervision.

The telemetry patient should be reassessed daily for the need to continue the telemetry monitoring. He or she should be visualized with each ECG alarm episode and clinically assessed. A daily skin assessment should be made to ensure that there is no skin breakdown or allergic reaction from the electrodes. Electrodes should be replaced daily. Ensure that appropriate alarm parameters are set based on the patient's condition. The battery should be checked daily and replaced as needed.

Common telemetry problems include loss of signal and artifact. Loss of signal can be due to:

- Battery problems, in which case the battery should be replaced.
- An electrode is loose or falling off, in which case the electrode should be replaced.
- The patient is taken off the monitor for transport to another area of the hospital, in which case the monitoring technician should be informed and the patient should be reattached to the monitor upon his or her return.

Artifact on the telemetry monitor frequently resolves with replacement and repositioning of the electrode.

TRANSTELEPHONIC CARDIAC MONITORING

Transtelephonic cardiac monitoring is an ambulatory ECG monitoring method that does not require the device to be worn continuously, but only during the phone monitoring period. This was initially devised for patients with pacemakers, but it has evolved for patients under evaluation for various arrhythmias. The patient is typically equipped with a finger electrode or a wrist bracelet attached to a monitor that acts as a transmitter to send heart rhythm data to the prescribing physician.

The patient is instructed to place the phone onto the transmitter, push the activation button, hold still, and wait while the data are transmitted to the cardiologist's office. The technician will assess for any symptoms and check that the data obtained are adequate. The patient is subsequently notified of the results. The quality of the data can be compromised by patient movement during the transmission. Additionally, if the patient lives in a remote area with poor phone reception, this can also compromise the monitoring attempts.

PERMANENT PACEMAKER

A permanent pacemaker is implanted to help maintain a regular heart rhythm when the patient's own signaling system is not functioning properly. The pacemaker is typically implanted under anesthesia via a skin incision in the left subclavian area, and wire leads are implanted into the right atrium and right ventricle. The leads attach to an implanted generator that contains a battery that monitors each heartbeat to ensure it is appropriate. If the patient's heart signaling system is too slow, the pacemaker will initiate a heartbeat to ensure that the patient does not become dizzy or fatigued or have a syncopal episode due to an abnormally slow heart rate. The pacemaker can be set to a variety of settings and thresholds depending on the patient's clinical scenario.

INSTRUCTIONS FOR PATIENTS UNDERGOING A PERMANENT PACEMAKER INSERTION

The patient undergoing pacemaker insertion should be informed that this a permanent device that will require routine follow-up with a cardiologist. Over time, the battery may run low, requiring a repeat procedure to replace it. Immediately following pacemaker insertion, the patient's left arm is usually placed in a sling to limit excessive movement and to lower the risk of pacemaker lead malposition. This assumes that the pacemaker is implanted in the left side of the chest of a right-handed patient because the nondominant side is the preferred implantation site. Similarly, the patient is instructed to avoid raising his or her left arm above the head to refrain from getting the incision area wet, and to watch for signs of redness or infection around the pacemaker site for at least 7–10 days postoperatively, at which time a follow-up office visit should occur. The patient should avoid electromagnetic radiation and magnetic resonance imaging (MRI) machines and should avoid using heavy electrical equipment, which can interfere with the pacemaker functioning.

TROUBLESHOOTING COMMON PACEMAKER PROBLEMS

Common pacemaker problems include failure to pace, in which case the patient's heart rate was slow enough that the pacemaker should have taken over and paced the patient's heart but did not. Causes for this can include lead fracture, lead displacement, or generator failure, and it may require a repeat procedure. Undersensing, in which the pacemaker does not detect that the patient's heart is producing its own signal and instead the pacemaker depolarizes inappropriately, can occur due to improper pacemaker programming, a lead fracture, or electrolyte problems. Finally, oversensing, in which the pacemaker inappropriately detects electrical signals and inhibits pacing, can occur due to electromagnetic interference or lead fracture. These problems should be assessed and corrected by the cardiologist.

AUTOMATED IMPLANTABLE CARDIOVERTER DEFIBRILLATOR (AICD)

The automated implantable cardioverter defibrillator (AICD) is a permanently implanted device in patients who have survived a cardiac arrest that did not have a reversible cause or as prophylactic therapy for patients who are at high risk for sudden cardiac death due to ventricular tachycardia (VT) or ventricular fibrillation due to a low left ventricular ejection fraction of <35%. One lead is implanted in the right atrium; the other is implanted in the right ventricle. The AICD can function as a pacemaker, preventing the heart rhythm from dropping too low. In addition, it can act as a cardioverter, attempting to pace the abnormal rhythm back to a normal rhythm. Most importantly, it can defibrillate the heart in the setting of a life-threatening ventricular arrhythmia, such as VT or ventricular fibrillation, thus internally delivering a painful yet effective shock to restore the normal heart rhythm.

INSTRUCTIONS FOR PATIENTS UNDERGOING AN AICD IMPLANTATION PROCEDURE

The patient undergoing an AICD implantation should be advised of the purpose of the procedure, namely, that the device will help prevent or terminate life-threatening ventricular arrhythmias. The patient will need to follow up with regular device checks in the physician's office and usually with a remote monitoring device set up at home as well. The battery lifespan and integrity of the leads are evaluated at routine office visits.

In the event of a device shock, the patient should contact the physician's office for further instructions. In the case of repetitive shocks, the patient should be evaluated immediately to determine whether the shocks were appropriate or inappropriate. In either case, further evaluation and testing may be warranted.

DETERMINATION OF THE APPROPRIATENESS OF AICD SHOCKS

In the case of repetitive shocks from the AICD, the first step is to have the device interrogated by a technician from the AICD company who will come to the hospital or office to perform this function. The interrogation provides graphics and data about the heart rhythms before, during, and after the shock in order to help determine if the shock was appropriate or inappropriate.

If the shock was appropriate, there was a life-threatening ventricular arrhythmia that occurred that was terminated by the device. Lab work including electrolytes, drug levels such as digoxin level, and possibly further cardiac testing should be performed to help assess if the patient's cardiac status has destabilized.

Inappropriate AICD shocks mean that the patient did not have a life-threatening arrhythmia but was shocked anyway. This needs to be corrected because it is a painful event for the patient and it puts excessive strain on the device's battery.

DEFIBRILLATORS

Common causes for inappropriate shocks include the following:

- Device malfunction—This can be caused by a fractured or dislodged lead. These are usually detected by chest x-ray and device interrogation, which assess the parameters of the lead function. The lead may need to be replaced or repositioned for complete resolution.
- Electromagnetic interference—This can confuse the defibrillator; some AICD devices prevent the patient from undergoing an MRI scan because the MRI creates noise that is sensed as a ventricular arrhythmia and can lead to shocks. Arc welding should also be avoided for the same reason.
- SVT—This can be mistaken for VT. It may be prevented by the addition of oral medication and, in some cases, radiofrequency ablation.

Performing Rhythm Analysis

Sinus Rhythm Data

SINUS BRADYCARDIA (SB)

There are 3 primary types of **sinus node dysrhythmias**: sinus bradycardia, sinus tachycardia, and sinus arrhythmia. **Sinus bradycardia (SB)** is caused by a decreased rate of impulse from sinus node. The pulse and ECG usually appear normal except for a slower rate.

SB is characterized by a regular pulse <50 to 60 with P waves in front of QRS, which are usually normal in shape and duration. PR interval is 0.12 to 0.20 seconds, QRS interval 0.04 to 0.11 seconds, and P:QRS ratio of 1:1. SB may be caused by a number of **factors**:

- Conditions that lower the body's metabolic needs, such as hypothermia or sleep.
- Hypotension and decrease in oxygenation.
- Medications such as calcium channel blockers and β-blockers.
- Vagal stimulation that may result from vomiting, suctioning, or defecating.
- Increased intracranial pressure.
- Myocardial infarction.

Treatment involves eliminating cause if possible, such as changing medications. Atropine 0.5-1.0 mg may be given IV to block vagal stimulation.

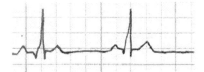
Sinus bradycardia

SINUS TACHYCARDIA (ST)

Sinus tachycardia (ST) occurs when the sinus node impulse increases in frequency. ST is characterized by a regular pulse >100 with P waves before QRS but sometimes part of the preceding T wave. QRS is usually of normal shape and duration (0.04 to 0.11 seconds) but may have consistent irregularity. PR interval is 0.12-0.20 seconds and P:QRS ratio of 1:1. The rapid pulse decreases diastolic filling time and causes reduced cardiac output with resultant hypotension. Acute pulmonary edema may result from the decreased ventricular filling if untreated. ST may be caused by a number of **factors**:

- Acute blood loss, shock, hypovolemia, anemia.
- Sinus arrhythmia, hypovolemic heart failure.
- Hypermetabolic conditions, fever, infection.

64

- Exertion/exercise, anxiety.
- Medications, such as sympathomimetic drugs.

Treatment includes eliminating precipitating factors and calcium channel blockers and β-blockers to reduce heart rate.

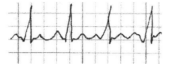 **Sinus tachycardia**

SINUS ARRHYTHMIA (SA)

Sinus arrhythmia (SA) results from irregular impulses from the sinus node, often paradoxical (increasing with inspiration and decreasing with expiration) because of stimulation of the vagal nerve during inspiration and rarely causes a negative hemodynamic effect. These cyclic changes in the pulse during respiration are quite common in both children and young adults and often lesson with age but may persist in some adults. Sinus arrhythmia can, in some cases, relate to heart or valvular disease and may be increased with vagal stimulation for suctioning, vomiting, or defecating. Characteristics of SA include a regular pulse 50-100 BPM, P waves in front of QRS with duration (0.04 to 0.11 seconds) and shape of QRS usually normal, PR interval of 0.12 to 0.20 seconds, and P:QRS ratio of 1:1. Treatment is usually not necessary unless it is associated with bradycardia.

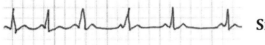 **Sinus arrhythmia**

CAUSES AND TREATMENTS OF ATRIAL FIBRILLATION

Atrial fibrillation is the most common abnormal heart rhythm. Causes can include the following:

- Increasing age
- Hypertension
- Coronary artery disease
- COPD
- Hyperthyroidism
- Heavy alcohol use

Treatment options depend on the patient's symptoms and on the duration of the atrial fibrillation. Common medications include oral or intravenous beta blockers or calcium channel blockers, which help control the heart rate, or antiarrhythmic medications such as sotalol, which can convert the rhythm to sinus.

In addition, direct-current cardioversion can be performed, and radiofrequency ablation can be considered in some cases. Finally, depending on the patient's risk profile, initiation of anticoagulation with oral blood thinners such as warfarin or apixaban can help reduce the risk of stroke.

SUPRAVENTRICULAR TACHYCARDIA (SVT)

Supraventricular tachycardia (SVT) is a commonly seen fast and regular heartbeat that originates in the atria, outside of the usual sinus node. The QRS complexes look narrow, but the P waves might be hard to see, or they occur just after the QRS complex. Episodes of SVT can occur suddenly. Typical symptoms include palpitations, dizziness, shortness of breath, or syncope. Triggers and causes can include psychological stress, alcohol, caffeine, illicit drugs, or thyroid problems. SVT is more common in females, especially during pregnancy, but it occurs in males as well. Episodes may be rare, and performing a vagal maneuver can usually slow down the heartbeat. If episodes are frequent, medications including calcium channel blockers such as diltiazem may be necessary. When episodes are frequent and severe, atrioventricular (AV) node radiofrequency ablation can be considered.

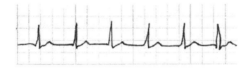 **Supraventricular tachycardia**

MULTIFOCAL ATRIAL TACHYCARDIA

Multifocal atrial tachycardia is a type of SVT. As such, the QRS complexes are narrow. The origin for the heartbeat is outside of the normal sinus node. The P waves have at least three different morphologies on display on the ECG. Each P wave is followed by a QRS complex. The heart rate is higher than 100 bpm. Multifocal atrial tachycardia is common in older patients with underlying conditions such as COPD, coronary artery disease, and congestive heart failure and in those recovering from surgery. Patients can have palpitations, shortness of breath, or have syncope. Treatment focuses on trying to correct the underlying cause and ensuring normal electrolyte balance. Medications that slow the heart, such as calcium channel blockers and beta blockers, are commonly used.

Atrial Rhythm Data

SEQUENCE OF ELECTRICAL DEPOLARIZATION OF A NORMAL HEARTBEAT

The signal for the heartbeat originates in the sinoatrial node, located in the upper right atrium near the superior vena cava. Then, the signal propagates to the left atrium as well, and both atria depolarize. After that, the signal travels downward to the atrioventricular (AV) node, located in the lower right atrium, near the tricuspid valve. There is a slightly prolonged propagation of the signal through the AV node (approximately 0.1 sec), allowing atrial contraction to be completed prior to the onset of ventricular depolarization. This allows the ventricles to fill with blood. Conduction fibers called the bundle of His then receive the depolarization, branching into the right and left bundle branches, which depolarize the interventricular septum. The signal then progresses to the Purkinje fibers, which terminate in the subendocardium of the right and left ventricles, causing ventricular contraction.

PREMATURE ATRIAL CONTRACTION (PAC)

There are 3 primary types of **atrial dysrhythmias**, including premature atrial contractions, atrial flutter, and atrial fibrillation. **Premature atrial contraction (PAC)** is essentially an extra beat precipitated by an electrical impulse to the atrium before the sinus node impulse. The extra beat may be caused by alcohol, caffeine, nicotine, hypervolemia, hypokalemia, hypermetabolic conditions, atrial ischemia or infarction. Characteristics include an irregular pulse because of extra P waves; shape and duration of QRS is usually normal (0.04 to 0.11 seconds) but may be abnormal, PR interval remains between 0.12 to 0.20, and P:QRS ratio is 1:1. Rhythm is irregular with varying P-P and R-R intervals. PACs can occur in an essentially healthy heart and are not usually cause for concern unless they are frequent (>6 hr) and cause severe palpitations. In that case, atrial fibrillation should be suspected.

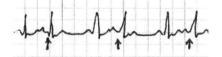

Premature atrial contraction

PHYSIOLOGICAL PROCESSES THAT OCCUR IN ATRIAL FIBRILLATION

Atrial fibrillation is classically described as an "irregularly irregular" rhythm with no identifiable P waves on the ECG. During the normal sinus rhythm, a single impulse for the heartbeat originates in the sinoatrial (SA) node of the right atrium, propagates to the left atrium, and moves through the AV node to the ventricles. In contrast, in atrial fibrillation, multiple sites in the atria send signals to the AV node, which result in chaotic and irregular depolarization of the ventricles. The QRS complexes have no identifiable regular rhythm.

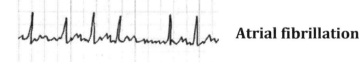

Atrial fibrillation

The presence of atrial fibrillation increases the risk of embolic stroke approximately five times compared to a patient in sinus rhythm. This is because the atria are quivering, rather than contracting fully with each heartbeat, making a blood clot more likely to form and flick off, which can lodge in the brain. The risk of stroke is increased whether the patient has chronic or intermittent atrial fibrillation. Patients may be started on blood thinners depending on their risk profile, thus lowering the risk of stroke.

ATRIAL FLUTTER VS. ATRIAL FIBRILLATION

Atrial flutter is classically described as a "sawtooth" pattern on ECG, with usually two to four P waves for every QRS. Commonly, the atrial rate is 300 bpm and the ventricular rate is 150 bpm. Atrial flutter is similar to atrial fibrillation in that it can cause symptoms such as palpitations, shortness of breath, or dizziness. Additionally, atrial flutter can increase the risk of ischemic stroke, and anticoagulation should be considered based on the patient's risk profile. The causes of atrial flutter are similar to those of atrial fibrillation. These include hypertension, coronary artery disease, COPD, hyperthyroidism, and heavy alcohol use. As for atrial fibrillation, treatment options include medications to slow the heart rate and cardioversion. Radiofrequency ablation is a frequently used treatment option.

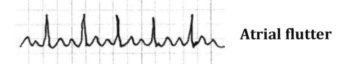 **Atrial flutter**

In contrast to atrial fibrillation, atrial flutter is a more organized rhythm, but it still represents disorganized atrial activity that is not sinus rhythm. It is less common than atrial fibrillation. Atrial flutter symptoms may be less severe than those of atrial fibrillation.

> **Review Video: EKG Interpretation: Atrial Fibrillation and Atrial Flutter**
> Visit mometrix.com/academy and enter code: 263842

Junctional Rhythm Data

JUNCTIONAL RHYTHMS

Junctional rhythm occurs when the electrical impulse for the heartbeat originates at or near the atrioventricular node instead of the sinoatrial node and then it depolarizes the ventricles. The usual heart rate is 40–60 bpm. Common causes of junctional rhythm include myocardial infarction, recent cardiac surgery, or digitalis toxicity.

Junctional rhythms have a regular R-R interval. The P waves may be absent; alternatively, the P waves may be inverted, reflecting backward conduction of the electrical impulse from the AV node toward the SA node.

An accelerated junctional rhythm has its origin in the AV node and a heart rate of 60–100 bpm, whereas a junctional tachycardia has its origin in the AV node and a heart rate of >100 bpm.

ECG DIAGNOSIS, SYMPTOMS, AND TREATMENT

Junctional rhythm has a narrow QRS complex, unless it is in the presence of RBBB or LBBB. Patients may notice lightheadedness, shortness of breath, or syncope. Treatment is directed at correcting the underlying condition, including electrolyte replacement and correction of digitalis toxicity. Discontinuing medications that slow the heart rate, including beta blockers, calcium channel blockers, or sotalol, may be necessary. In some cases, a permanent pacemaker or radiofrequency ablation may be considered.

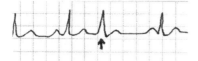

Premature junctional contractions

ECG DIAGNOSIS, CAUSES, AND TREATMENT OF ACCELERATED JUNCTIONAL RHYTHM

Accelerated junctional rhythm occurs when the rate of the AV junctional pacemaker beats exceeds the rate of the sinus node beats. The QRS complex is typically narrow unless a bundle block branch is present. The patient may experience shortness of breath or palpitations. The heart rate is 60–100 bpm. In contrast to SVT, this rhythm does not respond to vagal maneuvers. This rhythm can be irregular and display heart rate variability. Common causes include sick sinus syndrome, Lyme disease, and digitalis toxicity. Treatment is directed at the underlying cause and can include insertion of a permanent pacemaker. Digoxin toxicity is treated with the administration of Digibind (which binds the digoxin and eliminates it via the kidneys) or radiofrequency ablation.

Heart Block Rhythm Data

PHYSIOLOGIC PROCESS THAT THE PR INTERVAL REPRESENTS

The **PR interval** on the ECG represents the time from depolarization of the right and left atria (P wave) until depolarization of the ventricle (QRS complex), with the normal range being 0.120–0.20 sec (120–200 milliseconds, or up to one big box on the ECG tracing). Therefore, this interval effectively represents the atrioventricular conduction time, during which the electrical signal propagates from the atrium to the AV node and then to the bundle of His and the right and left bundle branches, which depolarizes the ventricles. A disruption of the normal PR interval can be a clue to disease: A shortened PR interval (of fewer than 120 msec) can indicate an arrhythmia, including Wolf–Parkinson–White syndrome, also called pre-excitation; a prolonged PR interval of greater than 200 msec represents first-degree AV block, which can be caused by certain medications and electrolyte abnormalities. Furthermore, if the PR interval is depressed below the baseline, it could indicate pericarditis.

ECG APPEARANCE OF FIRST-DEGREE AV BLOCK

In **first-degree AV block**, every QRS complex is preceded by a P wave, but the PR duration is greater than 0.20 seconds (longer than one big box on the ECG). The signal for depolarization is slower than normal because it travels from the atria through the AV node to the ventricles. Common causes can include medications such as beta blockers and conditions such as lupus, infectious diseases, myocarditis, enhanced vagal tone, and intrinsic atrioventricular node disease. In general, first-degree AV block is usually asymptomatic and does not require treatment.

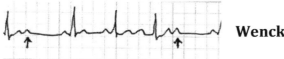

First-degree AV block

ECG Appearance of Type I Second-Degree Heart Block

In **type I second-degree heart block (Wenckebach rhythm)**, there is a progressive increase in the PR interval with each heartbeat until there is a P wave without a QRS following it. Therefore, this represents an intermittent failure of conduction through the AV node. The causes are similar to those of first-degree AV block, including drugs, vagal tone, infections such as myocarditis, or myocardial infarction. This is usually an asymptomatic condition with a benign prognosis. No specific treatment is needed in most cases.

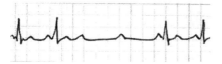

Wenckebach rhythm

The Wenckebach phenomenon was first noted in 1924 by Karel Wenckebach, a Dutch professor.

ECG of Type II Second-Degree AV Block

Type II second-degree AV block, or Mobitz II heart block, is a conduction problem located in the His-Purkinje system, which depolarizes the ventricles. On the ECG, there is a constant PR interval until there is a P wave but no QRS following it. Causes include myocardial infarction, amyloidosis, certain medications, inflammatory diseases such as sarcoidosis, and hyperkalemia. Patients may be hemodynamically unstable, have syncope, or be severely bradycardic. Importantly, this condition can progress to complete heart block. It warrants immediate medical attention, and it usually requires a pacemaker.

Type II second-degree AV block

Pathophysiology of Complete Heart Block

Third-degree AV block/complete heart block is a failure of the His-Purkinje system to conduct the electrical depolarization to the ventricles; the AV node does not conduct the atrial depolarization to the ventricles. The atria and ventricles beat independently of each other, with the atrial rate being faster than the ventricular rate. This rhythm is diagnosed when the P waves and QRS complexes are unrelated. The most common cause of complete heart block is coronary artery disease; however, infiltrative processes such as amyloidosis or medications should also be considered. Patients are typically profoundly bradycardic and can be dizzy or hemodynamically unstable. Patients usually require a pacemaker.

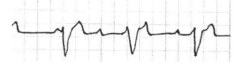 **Third-degree AV block**

FEATURES OF LBBB

LBBB is an ECG abnormality in which a block in the cardiac depolarization signal is blocked at the His-Purkinje level. Therefore, instead of a unified QRS deflection on ECG, in which the right and left ventricles are depolarized simultaneously, the right ventricle is first depolarized and then the signal propagates to the left ventricle. There is a slight delay as this occurs, and the QRS duration is >0.12 msec. Importantly, because of the LBBB morphology and its associated ST changes on ECG, myocardial infarction cannot be accurately diagnosed in the setting of LBBB by ECG alone because the baseline ECG of LBBB mimics ischemic changes. LBBB is associated with a higher risk of underlying cardiac abnormality, and, even if the patient is asymptomatic, this warrants cardiac testing. Treatment depends on the underlying cause, and it can include cardiac medications or a pacemaker.

RBBB and LBBB are similar in that both have QRS durations greater than 0.12 msec on ECG and they involve a bundle branch at the His-Purkinje level. Patients with either condition may be asymptomatic. Conversely, RBBB does not mimic ischemia on ECG, and it is usually a benign condition not requiring treatment, whereas LBBB precludes the diagnosis of myocardial infarction on ECG and it warrants further cardiac workup even if the patient is asymptomatic.

FEATURES OF RBBB

RBBB is an ECG abnormality in which the cardiac depolarization signal is blocked at the His-Purkinje level. Therefore, instead of a unified QRS deflection on ECG, in which the right and left ventricle are simultaneously depolarized, the left ventricle is first depolarized and then the signal propagates to the right ventricle. There is a slight delay as this occurs, resulting in the typical "M"-shaped morphology of the RBBB on ECG, and the QRS duration is >0.12 msec. Most patients are asymptomatic, and treatment is rarely necessary if the heart is structurally normal. However, some medical conditions carry an increased risk of RBBB, including COPD, pulmonary embolus, or myocardial infarction.

Ventricular Rhythm Data

VENTRICULAR TACHYCARDIA (VT)

Ventricular tachycardia (VT or V tach) is an abnormally fast heart rhythm in which the ventricles beat too fast to allow adequate filling of the chambers with

71

blood, with subsequent decreased oxygenation of the tissues. Heart rates are typically greater than 120 bpm. This can cause syncope, shortness of breath, palpitations, and even cardiac arrest. This condition can be due to scar tissue in the heart's conduction system, most commonly due to a prior heart attack. Myocarditis or heart valve disease are also possible causes. In the hemodynamically stable patient, VT is treated with medications, radiofrequency ablation, and in some cases implantation of an implantable cardioverter dcfibrillator. If the patient becomes severely symptomatic or hemodynamically unstable, defibrillation should be performed.

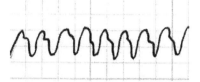 Ventricular tachycardia

> **Review Video: How to Identify Ventricular Arrhythmias on an EKG Strip**
> Visit mometrix.com/academy and enter code: 933152

PREMATURE VENTRICULAR CONTRACTIONS (PVCs)

A premature ventricular contraction (PVC) is a common but abnormal heartbeat that begins in the ventricle rather than in the atrium. It disrupts the normal heart rhythm and can feel like a fluttering sensation. A patient with frequent PVCs (comprising >20% of daily beats) could also experience palpitations, shortness of breath, or dizziness. PVCs are usually detected by Holter monitoring. The patient should undergo testing to exclude structural heart disease, including left ventricular hypertrophy, congestive heart failure, or coronary artery disease. Other causes include cardiac stimulants including excessive alcohol and caffeine consumption, which can irritate or stimulate the heart. Use of medications such as beta blockers and antiarrhythmics can be considered. Rarely, if the patient remains extremely symptomatic, PVC radiofrequency ablation may be necessary.

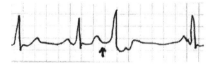 **Premature ventricular contraction**

IDIOVENTRICULAR RHYTHM

Ventricular escape rhythm (idioventricular) occurs when the Purkinje fibers below the AV node create an impulse. This may occur if the sinus node fails to fire or if there is blockage at the AV node so that the impulse does not go through. Idioventricular rhythm is characterized by a regular ventricular rate of 20-40 BPM. Rates >40 BPM are called accelerated idioventricular rhythm. The P wave is missing and the QRS complex has a very bizarre and abnormal shape with duration of ≥0.12 seconds. The low ventricular rate may cause a decrease in cardiac output, often making the patient lose consciousness. In other patients, the idioventricular rhythm may not be associated with reduced cardiac output.

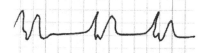 **Premature ventricular contraction**

Pacemaker Rhythm Data

NOMENCLATURE OF PACEMAKER FUNCTIONS

Pacemaker nomenclature is a code to describe antibradycardia pacemakers; it was established by the North American Society of Pacing and Electrophysiology and the British Pacing and Electrophysiology Group.

The pacemaker code has five positions:

X _ _ _ _ The chamber that is paced. It denotes the cardiac chamber in which the pacemaker stimulation occurs: O for none; A for atrium, V for ventricle, or D for both atrium and ventricle.

_ **X** _ _ _ The chamber sensed. It denotes the chamber in which the spontaneous cardiac depolarization can be detected: O for neither, A for atrium, V for ventricle, or D for both atrium and ventricle.

_ _ **X** _ _ Response to sensing. It describes the mode of response, whether a sensed event inhibits or triggers a response. I denotes inhibits, T denotes that a response is triggered, and D denotes that it both inhibits and triggers.

_ _ _ **X** _ Rate modulation. This refers to the automatic adjustment of the pacing rate to compensate for chronotropic incompetence. R denotes that this feature is present; O denotes that it is absent.

_ _ _ _ **X** Multisite pacing. It describes whether multisite pacing is present in each atrium or ventricle or in multiple stimulation sites: O denotes none, A denotes one or both atria, V denotes one or both ventricles, and D denotes any combination of atrium and ventricle.

DDDRO PACEMAKER

In a DDDRO pacemaker, there is an atrial lead and a ventricular lead. The first D refers to which heart chamber is paced—dual for both atrium and ventricle. The atrial lead will be triggered to pace the atrium if the native atrial heart rate falls below a threshold; this is commonly set at 60 bpm. In this case, a pacer spike will be seen as the atrium paces and depolarizes. The second D refers to which cardiac chamber is sensed by the pacemaker—again, dual, meaning both atrium and ventricle. The ventricle senses this atrial depolarization. If the native ventricle does not depolarize on its own, a ventricular pacing spike will be seen, followed by a wide QRS complex. The third D refers to what the pacemaker does in response to sensing,

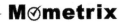

denoted as D for the ability to inhibit or to trigger. This type of pacemaker is commonly used for sick sinus syndrome or AV blocks. The R indicates that the unit includes rate modulation. The O denotes that there is no multisite pacing.

COMMON PACEMAKER MALFUNCTIONS

Some common pacemaker malfunctions and their causes include the following:

- Failure to output – There is an indication for pacing, but no pacing spike occurs. Its causes include battery failure or lead fracture.
- Failure to capture – There is a pacer spike, but it is not followed by an atrial or ventricular complex. Its causes include lead dislodgement or metabolic abnormalities such as hyperkalemia.
- Oversensing – The pacer is inhibited from correctly pacing due to oversensing electrical activity. Its causes include lead insulation breakage and muscular activity such as in the diaphragm or pectoralis muscle.
- Undersensing – Pacing occurs despite intrinsic depolarization. Its causes include poor lead positioning or a low battery level.

IMPORTANT INFORMATION TO KNOW UPON PACEMAKER INSERTION

After pacemaker implantation, the patient should be advised that he or she will need regular monitoring of the device, both remotely and in person. The cardiologist implanting the pacemaker will usually set up a home monitoring machine that will remotely download and transmit pacemaker data and allow for remote analysis of the heart rhythm. The patient will usually require in-person office visits every 6 to 12 months to check the battery life, test the pacemaker, and make adjustments if necessary. The patient should carry a wallet card listing the date of pacemaker implantation and the company name of the device. He or she should be advised not to push or twist the generator under the skin surface. There should be no problem with microwaves or TV remote controls interfering with the pacemaker. Depending on the device, the pacemaker may interfere with obtaining an MRI scan; the cardiologist can advise on the safety of this test depending on the specific device implanted.

Obtained Rhythm Data

BASIC FRAMEWORK FOR COMMUNICATING RHYTHM DATA

In analysis of rhythm issues, one should first ascertain if there are upright P waves and then assess the QRS complex.

Assessing rhythm data with an absent or fluttering P wave:

P Wave	QRS Complex	QRS Complex >0.12 sec	Rhythm Regularity	Diagnosis
Absent	Absent	No	No	Ventricular fibrillation or asystole
Absent	Present	Yes	Yes	Ventricular tachycardia
Absent	Present	No	None	Atrial fibrillation
Fluttering	Present	No	Sawtooth	Atrial flutter

Assessing rhythm data with the P wave present:

QRS with P Wave	PR Interval >0.20 sec	Diagnosis
No	No	Third-degree AV block
Intermittently	Possibly	Second-degree AV block
Yes	Yes	First-degree AV block
Yes	No	Normal sinus rhythm

ECG Findings

WAVEFORMS AS DEPOLARIZATION PROGRESSES FROM THE ATRIA TO THE VENTRICLES

The signal for heartbeat formation originates in the atrium and progresses to the ventricle:

- The P wave corresponds to atrial depolarization. It is a smooth upright bump with a positive deflection in lead II, with a duration of up to 0.11 seconds.
- The Q wave signifies ventricular septal depolarization. The Q wave is a negative deflection preceding the R wave. Q waves can be normal in some leads. However, pathologic Q waves can indicate a current or prior myocardial infarction. Features of pathologic Q waves include the following: width >1 mm, depth >2 mm, or >25% of the depth of the QRS complex. Q waves in leads V1–V3 are also considered pathologic.
- The R wave represents depolarization of the base of the ventricles. The size of the R wave should increase across the precordium. Absence of the R wave could hint to myocardial infarction. Conversely, a tall R wave in V1 can be a sign of various conditions, including RBBB, hypertrophic cardiomyopathy, and posterior myocardial infarction.
- The S wave is the first negative deflection after the R wave. When present, it typically is largest in V1 and decreases in size across the precordium. Its presence or absence is usually not clinically significant.

75

- The T wave denotes ventricular repolarization. The T wave is usually a positive deflection in most leads, following the positive deflection of its preceding QRS complex. When T waves are negative or inverted with ST segment depression or elevation, this is concerning for myocardial infarction or ischemia.
- The U wave is sometimes seen following the T wave. It represents Purkinje fiber repolarization.

SEGMENTS ON ECG

The term "segment" on ECG refers to the region between two waves.

- The PR segment represents the conduction of the cardiac impulse from the atria to the ventricles. The PR segment starts at the end of the P wave and ends with the start of the QRS complex. PR segment depression from the isoelectric line can help diagnose pericarditis.
- The ST segment starts at the end of the QRS wave and ends at the start of the T wave. It represents the beginning of ventricular repolarization. It is usually isoelectric. ST-segment analysis forms the basis for diagnosis of myocardial ischemia and infarction.
- The TP segment starts at the end of the T wave and the start of the next P wave. This represents the true isoelectric segment of the ECG, during which the heart is electrically silent.

INTERVALS ON ECG

An interval is a duration of time that includes one segment and one or more waves:

- The PR interval starts at the beginning of the P wave (which is the onset of atrial depolarization), and it ends with the start of the QRS complex (which is the onset of ventricular depolarization). The normal PR interval is 120–200 msec. The PR interval is lengthened in cases of first-degree AV block.
- The QRS interval is the total time of ventricular depolarization, usually 60–100 msec. The QRS interval is prolonged in cases of bundle branch block.
- The RR interval is the distance between two consecutive R waves. It should be constant if the patient is in normal sinus rhythm.
- The QT interval represents electrical ventricular systole, that is, ventricular depolarization and repolarization. The normal duration is 240–450 msec. Short or long QT intervals can be genetic in nature and predispose a patient to life-threatening ventricular arrhythmias, including torsades de pointes and ventricular fibrillation. A long QT interval can also be due to certain medications such as hydroxychloroquine and some antipsychotics. Other conditions such as hypothyroidism and hypokalemia can also prolong the QT interval.

Life-Threatening Arrhythmias

PULSELESS VT, VENTRICULAR FIBRILLATION, AND ASYSTOLE

Three of the most commonly encountered life-threatening arrhythmias are pulseless VT, ventricular fibrillation, and asystole. The ability to quickly identify and treat them is a life-saving skill.

Pulseless VT, an abnormal heart rhythm in which the ventricles are beating too quickly to properly perfuse the body, is a medical emergency requiring cardiopulmonary resuscitation (CPR) and shock with a defibrillator. If not terminated, it frequently progresses to ventricular fibrillation.

Ventricular fibrillation is the common cause of sudden cardiac arrest. There is no cardiac output, and the patient will die if this rhythm is not reversed. Treatment includes CPR and shock with a defibrillator.

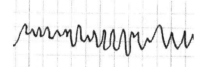 **Ventricular fibrillation**

Asystole looks like a flatline on ECG. It is treated with CPR and intravenous epinephrine. It is not a shockable rhythm. The underlying cause should be identified and reversed if possible.

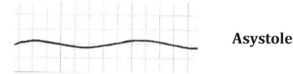 **Asystole**

Types of Artifact

CAUSES OF ARTIFACT ON ECG

The ability to identify artifact on ECG is important because it can mimic life-threatening arrhythmias such as VT and atrial fibrillation. In some cases, artifact can be easily suspected, such as when the patient remains hemodynamically stable despite a dramatically abnormal looking ECG. Similarly, an unstable or shaky baseline on ECG before, during, or after the episode of arrhythmia is also suspicious for artifact.

Other common causes of artifact on ECG include tremor, movement or shaking by the patient, electrical interference, a loose wire, lead misplacement, or medical devices commonly used on patients in operating rooms or intensive care units.

Classes/Effects of General Cardiovascular Medications

CALCIUM CHANNEL BLOCKERS

Calcium channel blockers, or calcium channel antagonists, inhibit the transport of calcium across cell membranes of the myocardium of the heart and vascular muscles, leading to the dilation or widening of the vasculature. This, in turn, increases the delivery of blood and oxygen to the heart, decreasing the heart's workload. The net result of calcium channel blockade is a decrease in blood pressure. The calcium channel blockers are divided into two classes: dihydropyridines and non-dihydropyridines. Verapamil and diltiazem, non-dihydropyridines, also lead to a decrease in heart rate. The remaining calcium channel blockers, specifically nifedipine, may cause an increase in heart rate.

Calcium channel blockers are used to treat high blood pressure, attacks of chest pain, and some arrhythmias. All the calcium channel blockers exhibit similar effectiveness in treating high blood pressure, but they exert their activity at different sites on the calcium channel receptors. Common side effects of the dihydropyridines include overall weakness, dizziness, headache, flushing, heartburn, or swelling of the extremities. Non-dihydropyridines, verapamil and diltiazem, may cause loss of appetite, nausea, low blood pressure, and swelling of the extremities. Verapamil has also been shown to cause constipation. Calcium channel blockers are commonly administered orally, but may be given intravenously in certain cases.

> **Review Video: Calcium Channel Blockers**
> Visit mometrix.com/academy and enter code: 942825

NITRATES

Nitrates are a class of cardiac medications used to decrease the heart's oxygen demand. The drugs relax the muscles in the blood vessels, allowing them to widen. By relaxing the coronary arteries, the workload on the heart is diminished, meaning the heart does not need to work as hard to pump blood to the body. By relaxing the blood vessels and allowing them to dilate, nitrates lead to a decrease in blood pressure. Often, use of nitrates may lead to an increased heart rate or tachycardia, but they may also cause a slowing of the heart rate, or bradycardia, in some instances. The class of nitrates includes drugs such as isosorbide mononitrate, isosorbide dinitrate, and nitroglycerin.

Nitrates, including drugs such as isosorbide mononitrate, isosorbide dinitrate, and nitroglycerin, are used to treat acute attacks of chest pain, or angina, prevent stress-induced attacks of chest pain, or for long-term prophylaxis of chest pain. For long-term use, nitrates are usually administered in combination with a beta-blocker or calcium channel blocker. Depending on the indication, nitrates are available for administration by several pathways. For rapid termination of an acute attack, nitrates may be administered via the sublingual or buccal pathway. Oral and transdermal formulations are available for prevention of chest pain or long-term use. Common side effects of the nitrates include dizziness, headache, lightheadedness, increased pulse, flushing of the head or neck, nausea or vomiting, and restlessness.

CARDIAC GLYCOSIDES

Cardiac glycosides are naturally occurring chemicals and include the drugs digoxin and digitoxin. These drugs bind to the sodium-potassium-ATP pump in the membranes of the cells of the myocardium. This leads to a decrease in the outflow of sodium from cardiac cells, causing a buildup of intracellular sodium. The increased sodium concentration slows the sodium-calcium exchange across the cell membrane, leading to a subsequent increase in the intracellular concentration of calcium. The increased calcium within the cardiac cells causes an increased force of contraction with each heartbeat. With the increased force, each heartbeat is stronger, pumping more blood. This, in turn, causes the heart to beat slower and stronger. While cardiac glycosides lower the heart rate, they have no appreciable effect on blood pressure. Digoxin also has a direct effect on arrhythmias by decreasing the conduction of electrical impulses through the atrioventricular node and prolonging the refractory period.

BETA BLOCKERS

Beta blockers are a widely used group of cardiac medications that block norepinephrine and epinephrine (adrenaline) from binding to beta receptors in the body. In doing this, they lower the heart rate and lower the blood pressure. Examples of beta blockers include atenolol, carvedilol, and metoprolol.

Common side effects of beta blockers include fatigue, bradycardia, heart block, shortness of breath, erectile dysfunction, and altered glucose metabolism. If a beta blocker is suddenly discontinued, it can cause rebound tachycardia or hypertension that can be difficult to control.

ANGIOTENSIN-CONVERTING ENZYME (ACE) INHIBITORS

Angiotensin-converting enzyme (ACE) inhibitors are a group of cardiac medications that block the formation of the blood pressure-regulating hormone angiotensin I into angiotensin II. Angiotensin II is a strong vasoconstrictor, which acts to raise blood pressure. When the conversion of angiotensin I to angiotensin II is blocked, blood pressure is better controlled. Examples of ACE inhibitors include lisinopril, enalapril, and ramipril.

Common side effects of ACE inhibitors include dry cough, hyperkalemia, and elevated creatinine. ACE inhibitors are contraindicated in any stage of pregnancy due to the risk of birth defects.

VAUGHAN WILLIAMS CLASSES OF ANTIARRHYTHMIC DRUGS

Antiarrhythmic drugs affect the electrical conduction through the heart, thereby helping to control the heart rhythm through a variety of mechanisms to reduce symptoms. The **Vaughan Williams classification** provides a framework for distinguishing these drugs:

- Class I, or sodium channel blockers, including flecainide.
- Class II, or beta blockers, including propranolol.
- Class III drugs such as amiodarone work through potassium channel blockade, prolonging the action potential and refractory period.
- Class IV, or calcium channel blockers, including verapamil.
- Class V including miscellaneous drugs, such as adenosine and digoxin, whose mechanism of action does not fit into classes I–IV.

Image Credits

https://en.wikipedia.org/wiki/Hexaxial_reference_system#/media/File:Hexaxial_reference_system.svg [public domain]

CCT Practice Test

1. Which heart chamber functions to pump deoxygenated blood to the lungs?

    a. Right atrium
    b. Right ventricle
    c. Left atrium
    d. Left ventricle

2. Which lead is the most affected by respiration?

    a. V2
    b. V4
    c. Lead III
    d. Lead I

3. Which of the following is the correct sequence by which action potentials are conducted through the heart?

    a. SA node → AV node → bundle branches → Purkinje fibers
    b. Bundle branches → Purkinje fibers → SA node → AV node
    c. Purkinje fibers → SA node → bundle branches → AV node
    d. AV node → SA node → bundle branches → Purkinje fibers

4. What type of heart block is seen in the following electrocardiogram (ECG) strip?

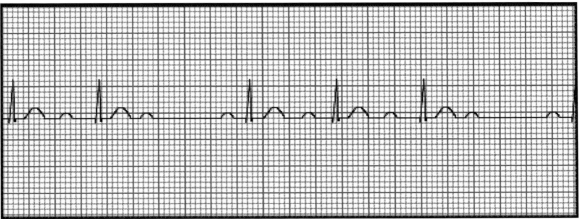

    a. First-degree heart block
    b. Second-degree heart block, type 1
    c. Second-degree heart block, type 2
    d. Third-degree heart block

5. When calibrating an ECG machine, what is the standard size of the calibration mark representing the sensitivity of the ECG machine?

a. 5 mm in height
b. 10 mm in height
c. 15 mm in height
d. 20 mm in height

6. Which of the following is the mechanism of action of nitrates?

a. Decrease the responsiveness of heart to the sympathetic nervous system
b. Lower the heart rate
c. Decrease cardiac contractility
d. Dilation of coronary arteries

7. Which phase of the action potential in fast response myocardial tissues consists of rapid depolarization, with the resting cell being brought to threshold?

a. Phase 0
b. Phase 1
c. Phase 2
d. Phase 3

8. The depolarizing current in pacemaker cells is created primarily by which of the following ions?

a. Sodium
b. Calcium
c. Potassium
d. Chloride

9. Which of the following commonly limits the diagnostic value of Holter monitoring?

a. Patient noncompliance with keeping track of events
b. Lack of continuous monitoring
c. Small capacity of recording devices
d. Transmission of data depends on patient participation

10. Which of the following effects is caused by the actions of the parasympathetic nervous system on the heart?

a. Increased rate of conduction
b. Greater force of contraction
c. Decreased diastolic filling time
d. Decreased rate of SA node pacing

11. What does the T wave represent on an ECG?

a. Atrial depolarization
b. Ventricular depolarization
c. Atrial repolarization
d. Ventricular repolarization

12. What benefit does a thallium stress test have as compared to a standard ECG stress test?

a. More quickly identifies areas of myocardial ischemia in the heart
b. The test is simpler to perform
c. More accurately identifies the specific areas of reduced blood flow in the heart
d. Is a safer test overall for the patient

13. Which of the following is the correct placement of chest leads for a 12-lead ECG?

a. V1 in the third intercostal space, immediately right of the sternum. V2 in the fourth intercostal space, immediately left of the sternum. V3 midway between V2 and V4. V4 in the fifth intercostal space, at the midclavicular line. V5 in the fourth intercostal space, at the anterior axillary line. V6 in the third intercostal space, at the midaxillary line.
b. V1 in the fourth intercostal space, immediately right of the sternum. V2 in the fifth intercostal space, immediately right of the sternum. V3 in the fifth intercostal space, immediately left of the sternum. V4 in the fifth intercostal space, at the midclavicular line. V5 in the fifth intercostal space, at the anterior axillary line. V6 in the fifth intercostal space, at the midaxillary line.
c. V1 in the fourth intercostal space, immediately right of the sternum. V2 in the fourth intercostal space, immediately left of the sternum. V3 midway between V2 and V4. V4 in the sixth intercostal space, directly below V2. V5 in the fifth intercostal space, at the midclavicular line. V6 in the fourth intercostal space, at the midaxillary line.
d. V1 in the fourth intercostal space, immediately right of the sternum. V2 in the fourth intercostal space, immediately left of the sternum. V3 midway between V2 and V4. V4 in the fifth intercostal space, at the midclavicular line. V5 in the fifth intercostal space, at the anterior axillary line. V6 in the fifth intercostal space, at the midaxillary line.

14. How many leaflets does the mitral valve have?

a. One
b. Two
c. Three
d. Four

15. What is being measured when determining the height or depth of a wave from the baseline on an ECG?

    a. Power
    b. Current
    c. Voltage
    d. Resistance

16. What is the most likely cause of the vertical, upwards spikes seen in the ECG strip below?

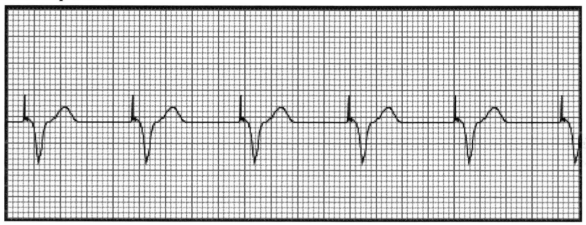

    a. Pacemaker firing
    b. Spontaneous AV node firing
    c. ECG leads placed too closely together
    d. Heart block

17. Which of the following is NOT an indication for Holter monitoring?

    a. Assessing pacemaker function
    b. Evaluating syncopal episodes
    c. Assessing for ischemia
    d. Evaluating for a new infarction

18. What is the difference between the first stage of the "Bruce protocol" stress test and the first stage of the "Modified Bruce protocol" stress test?

    a. The Modified Bruce protocol starts at the same gradient, but at a slower speed for the first stage of the test.
    b. The Modified Bruce protocol starts at the same speed, but at a lower gradient for the first stage of the test.
    c. The Modified Bruce protocol starts at a lower gradient and a slower speed for the first stage of the test.
    d. There is no difference between the first stage of the two protocols.

19. A patient is found to have a normal heart rate and rhythm. It is determined from an ECG that the axis of the heart is -35°. What does this indicate?

    a. The heart is in its normal axis range
    b. The patient has vertical axis deviation
    c. The patient has right axis deviation
    d. The patient has left axis deviation

20. Which of the following skin preparations should be done before Holter monitor electrode placement?

    a. Abrasion of the skin
    b. Removal of all chest hair
    c. Disinfection of the skin
    d. Moisturization of the skin

21. Where is the sinoatrial node located?

    a. Medial part of left atrium
    b. Posterior part of right atrium
    c. Superior part of left atrium
    d. Inferior part of right atrium

22. When the ECG below was performed, what was done incorrectly by the ECG technician?

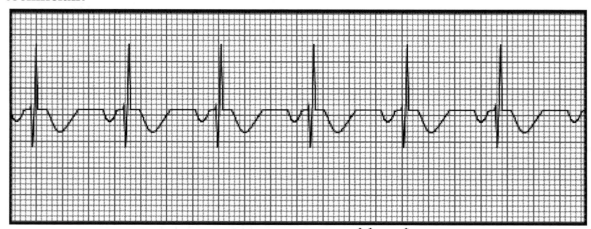

    a. The machine was not calibrated correctly
    b. The paper in the machine was placed upside down
    c. The placement of the leads was reversed
    d. The precordial leads and limb leads were intermixed

23. At what level above baseline should ST segment elevation begin to be considered abnormal?

    a. 0 mm
    b. 1 mm
    c. 4 mm
    d. 6 mm

24. When narrow QRS complexes appear earlier than expected on a Holter tracing, but otherwise appear identical to the sinus complexes, what is the likely diagnosis?

a. Junctional extrasystole
b. Premature supraventricular beats
c. Atrial flutter
d. Premature ventricular beats

25. The period during which a cell will not respond to action potentials transmitted from other cells is referred to as the _____.

a. unresponsive period.
b. effectual limiting period.
c. depolarization control period.
d. effective refractory period.

26. If a patient's heart rate suddenly drops to 40 beats per minute (bpm) and he becomes acutely confused and ill, what medication should be given first?

a. Dopamine
b. Sotalol
c. Epinephrine
d. Atropine

27. In which individuals is spontaneous fluctuation in the PR interval most often seen?

a. Individuals with normal hearts
b. Individuals on beta-blockers
c. Individuals with an AV nodal bypass track
d. Individuals with an AV block

28. In order for an exercise stress test to be adequate, the patient must reach what percentage of his or her age-predicted maximum heart rate?

a. 65%
b. 75%
c. 85%
d. 95%

29. The right and left coronary arteries branch off of which blood vessel?

a. Ascending aorta
b. Descending aorta
c. Pulmonary artery
d. Posterior descending artery

30. What type of rhythm is seen in the following ECG strip?

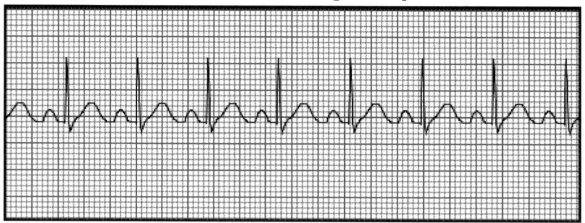

   a. Normal sinus rhythm
   b. Sinus tachycardia
   c. Supraventricular tachycardia
   d. Atrial flutter

31. Which of the following would be LEAST likely to complicate the diagnosis of myocardial ischemia based on Holter monitor tracings?
   a. If the patient has atrial fibrillation
   b. If the patient has a left bundle branch block
   c. If the patient is on digoxin
   d. If the patient is on a beta-blocker

32. Which cardiac cells have the fastest rate of spontaneous depolarization?
   a. Cells of the AV node
   b. Cells of the SA node
   c. Cells of the Purkinje fiber network
   d. Cells of the bundle branches

33. What is the term used to described the ventricular volume at the end of diastole?
   a. Preload
   b. Stroke volume
   c. Afterload
   d. End-systolic volume

34. If bradycardia during atrial fibrillation is observed on the Holter tracing, what type of problem does this likely indicate?
   a. A problem with ventricular depolarization
   b. A sinoatrial node problem
   c. An atrioventricular conduction problem
   d. Decreased sympathetic nervous system stimulation

35. Under what conditions might you expect to see consistent and diffuse low amplitude on an ECG?

   a. In an obese patient
   b. In a patient with congestive heart failure
   c. In a very athletic patient
   d. In a patient with a recent myocardial infarction

36. What is the normal resting potential of most myocardial cells?

   a. Between 0 and 10 mV
   b. Between 20 and 45 mV
   c. Between 80 and 95 mV
   d. Between 100 and 120 mV

37. Which of the following is the correct sequence for cardiac blood flow?

   a. Vena cava → left atrium → mitral valve → left ventricle → pulmonary valve→ pulmonary artery → lungs → pulmonary vein → right atrium → tricuspid valve → right ventricle → aortic valve → aorta
   b. Vena cava → right atrium → mitral valve → right ventricle → pulmonary valve → pulmonary artery → lungs → pulmonary vein → left atrium → tricuspid valve→ left ventricle → aortic valve → aorta
   c. Vena cava → right atrium → tricuspid valve → right ventricle → pulmonary valve → pulmonary artery → lungs → pulmonary vein → left atrium → mitral valve→ left ventricle → aortic valve → aorta
   d. Vena cava → left atrium → mitral valve → left ventricle → aortic valve → right atrium → tricuspid valve → right ventricle → pulmonary valve→ pulmonary artery → lungs

38. What precautions should be taken to avoid electric shock of the patient when performing an ECG?

   a. Make sure the patient is directly connected to a ground
   b. Ensure that the chassis is grounded
   c. Make sure the patient is connected to monitoring equipment that provides a direct connection to ground
   d. Avoid the use of line isolation transformers

39. Which of the following would be more likely to indicate a supraventricular tachycardia as opposed to a ventricular tachycardia on a Holter tracing?

   a. Heart rate of 200 bpm
   b. QRS complex of greater than 140 msec
   c. Monomorphic QRS complexes
   d. Very slight prematurity of the first complex

40. What is the group of cardiac cells that transmit electrical impulses from the AV node to the ventricles called?

    a. Sinoatrial node
    b. Intraventricular septum
    c. Bundle of His
    d. Purkinje fibers

41. What is often the first sign of digitalis toxicity on ECG?

    a. Premature ventricular contractions
    b. Ventricular fibrillation
    c. Premature atrial contractions
    d. Atrial flutter

42. Which of the following is a contraindication for stress testing?

    a. Patient is unable to exercise
    b. Complete left bundle branch block
    c. Acute pericarditis
    d. Coronary artery disease

43. Identify the abnormality seen in the ECG below.

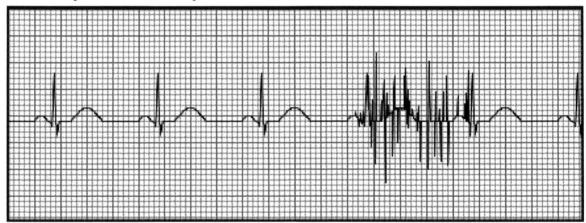

    a. Atrial flutter
    b. Transient supraventricular tachycardia
    c. Ventricular fibrillation
    d. Muscle tremor

44. Which of the following is appropriate electrode placement with ambulatory ECG monitors?

    a. Four electrodes are placed on the trunk
    b. Five electrodes are placed on the trunk, and one electrode is placed on each shoulder
    c. Five or more electrodes are placed on the trunk
    d. Six electrodes are placed on the trunk, one electrode is placed on the left upper thigh, and one electrode is placed on each shoulder

45. Which of the following activities should the patient avoid while the Holter monitor is in use?

a. Yard work
b. Sex
c. Showering
d. Running

46. Which of the following describes what would classically be seen on ECG if a patient has atrial flutter?

a. A rapid run of identical, consecutive waves that mask the baseline and are interspersed with QRS complexes
b. Continuous chaotic spikes that mask the baseline along with irregularly interspersed QRS complexes
c. Normal appearing sequences of P waves and QRS complexes that occur at a much faster rate than normal
d. A rapid series of waves of similar amplitude appearing as a smooth, wavy line

47. How are cardiac cells able to depolarize spontaneously and thus demonstrate automaticity?

a. They are consistently triggered by the sympathetic nervous system
b. They have an unstable resting potential that allows influx of calcium and sodium
c. They have increased permeability to potassium ions while in a resting state
d. Parasympathetic nervous system fibers regularly trigger the cells

48. Which class of antiarrhythmic agents act by blocking sodium channels?

a. Class I
b. Class II
c. Class III
d. Class IV

49. Movement of the Holter monitor cable can result in artifact on the recording, which may appear as movements of the baseline. Movement of the baseline would make it especially difficult to interpret what part of the recording?

a. QT length changes
b. QRS complex abnormalities
c. PR interval lengthening
d. ST segment changes

50. Which of the following agents is NOT typically used for pharmacologic stress testing?

a. Dipyridamole
b. Dobutamine
c. Adenosine
d. Norepinephrine

Answer Key and Explanations

1. B: The right ventricle pumps the deoxygenated blood it has received from the right atrium to the lungs. The right atrium pumps deoxygenated blood from the body to the right ventricle. The left atrium pumps oxygenated blood from the lungs to the left ventricle. The left ventricle pumps oxygenated blood to the body.

2. C: Lead III is the most affected by respiration, and therefore the waveforms may look different depending on the respiratory cycle. Because of this, a Q wave that *only* appears in lead III and is not associated with other corresponding changes in other leads is not significant.

3. A: The sequence by which an action potential is conducted through the heart is from the sinoatrial (SA) node to the atrioventricular (AV) node to the bundle branches and then to the Purkinje fibers.

4. B: The pictured ECG is a second-degree heart block, type 1. This rhythm is also called Mobitz I or Wenckebach. With this heart block the PR interval gets longer with each beat until eventually a P wave occurs, but a QRS does not follow (a beat is skipped). After the skipped beat, the pattern starts over again. A first-degree heart block occurs when the PR interval is longer than 0.2 seconds, but the PR interval generally remains constant and the QRS is not dropped. A second-degree heart block, type 2, also called Mobitz II, is apparent when the QRS suddenly fails to show up after a P wave. A fairly consistent ratio of P waves to QRS complexes is common, and this rhythm lacks the increasing PR interval that is seen in the Mobitz I block. A third-degree heart block is also called a complete heart block and the atria and ventricles beat independently of one another.

5. B: The calibration mark representing the sensitivity of the ECG should be 10 mm in height (two large squares). This mark is usually found on the left side of the page at the beginning of each line of the ECG. When this is set correctly it means that for every millivolt measured from the patient, a deflection of 10 mm will be recorded on the trace.

6. D: Nitrates are useful for the prevention and treatment of angina. They work by dilating the coronary arteries and thus increasing the blood flow to the heart. They dilate peripheral veins, and, in higher doses, other peripheral arteries, which decreases preload and afterload. Beta-blockers decrease the responsiveness of the heart to the sympathetic nervous system. Calcium channel blockers, beta-blockers, and other medications decrease cardiac contractility and decrease heart rate.

7. A: Phase 0 consists of rapid depolarization of the cell to threshold, which leads to activation of voltage-dependent sodium channels. Phase 1 consists of a slight "notch" of repolarization caused mainly by the activation of transient potassium currents (potassium leaving the cell) and a corresponding rapid decrease in the sodium current. Phase 2 is a plateau phase during which "late" calcium, and to a

93

lesser extent sodium, currents offset the effect of potassium currents and temporarily stabilize the membrane potential. Phase 3 refers to repolarization and return to resting potential due to increased potassium currents. Phase 4 is the resting membrane potential.

8. B: The depolarizing current in cardiac pacemaker cells is carried primarily by relatively slow, inward calcium currents. In most other depolarizing cells, such as muscle cells, the depolarization is created by fast sodium currents. Potassium plays a role in repolarization of the cells.

9. A: Patient noncompliance with keeping a diary of their symptoms and using event markers significantly limits the diagnostic value of Holter monitoring. It is important for patients to record and mark their symptoms in order to correlate events with the data collected. Holter monitoring is a type of continuous monitoring and benefits include the large capacity of the recording devices as well as the ability to transmit data without patient participation.

10. D: The parasympathetic nervous system results in cardiac inhibitory effects, including decreased rate of SA node pacing, decreased rate of conduction, and decreased force of contraction. The sympathetic nervous system increases the rate of conduction and causes increased force of contraction. An increased contraction rate, caused by sympathetic nervous system stimulation, would result in decreased diastolic filling time.

11. D: Repolarization of the ventricles begins immediately after the QRS. The T wave represents the final and more rapid phase of that repolarization. Atrial depolarization is represented by the P wave. Ventricular depolarization is represented by the QRS complex. Atrial repolarization is not seen on the ECG.

12. C: Thallium stress tests, also known as nuclear stress tests, gather more specific and accurate information than simple ECG stress tests. It is a helpful test when trying to identify the severity of coronary artery disease in a patient with known coronary disease.

13. D: The appropriate placement of the chest leads is very important for obtaining an accurate ECG. In order to determine whether the electrical activity of the heart is normal or abnormal, and to determine more precisely what type abnormality is present, it is necessary for these leads to be placed precisely and consistently. V1 and V2 are oriented over the right side of the heart, V3 and V4 are oriented over the interventricular septum, and V5 and V6 are oriented over the left side of the heart.

14. B: The mitral valve is a bicuspid valve, meaning that it has two leaflets (also known as cusps). It is located between the left atrium and left ventricle. The tricuspid valve, located between the right atrium and right ventricle, has three leaflets. The pulmonic valve leads from the right ventricle to the pulmonary artery and has three leaflets. The aortic valve leads from the left ventricle to the aorta and normally has three leaflets.

15. C: The amplitude of waves as measured from the baseline is a measure of voltage. Voltage is also known as electrical potential difference, and therefore gives us a picture of the depolarization and repolarization of the heart. These measurements are made in millimeters.

16. A: These spikes are an artifact due to the firing of an implanted pacemaker. In the above ECG the pacemaker is firing at regular intervals and each spike is followed by a QRS complex and a T wave. This is a normal ECG for a patient with a firing implanted pacemaker.

17. D: Holter (ambulatory) ECG monitoring can be useful in evaluating cardiac rhythm abnormalities, assessing pacemaker and implantable defibrillator function, assessing for ischemia, and evaluating heart rate variability. Ambulatory ECGs can be used to rule out conditions that may be missed on routine ECGs. Evaluation for an infarction should be done as an inpatient care since this requires immediate treatment if a new infarction is present.

18. B: Stage 1 of the Bruce protocol is a speed of 1.7 mph and gradient of 10%; stage 2 is a speed of 2.5 mph and a gradient of 12%. Stage 1 of the Modified Bruce protocol is a speed of 1.7 mph and a gradient of 0%; stage 2 is a speed of 1.7 mph and a 5% grade. The third stage of the Modified Bruce protocol corresponds to the first stage of the standard Bruce protocol and continues on from there. The Modified Bruce protocol is typically used for elderly or sedentary patients.

19. D: The normal axis of the heart is between 0° and +90°, which is downwards and to the left. If the axis is upwards and to the left (between 0° and -90°), that is considered left axis deviation. If the axis is to the right (between +90° and -90°), it is considered right axis deviation.

20. A: Abrading the thin outer layer of skin helps the electrodes adhere better to the skin, making them less likely to lose contact. The electrodes are also taped to the skin. If a patient has an especially hairy chest, the chest hair may need to be clipped in order to allow for proper adherence, but removal of all chest hair is not necessary. Disinfection and moisturization are not typical steps in skin preparation.

21. B: The SA node is located in the posterior wall of the right atrium, near the entrance of the superior vena cava. The AV node is located in the inferior region of the right atrium.

22. C: This patient has a normal rate and rhythm, but the appearance of the ECG is abnormal because the leads have been reversed. Reversal of lead placement has led to an ECG strip with negative (inverted) P waves, QRS complexes, and T waves. This is a common mistake when placing ECG leads and can lead to confusion when reading the ECG.

23. B: The ST segment should be isoelectric, meaning that it is level with the baseline. ST elevation is above 1 mm (or 0.1 mV) above baseline in a limb lead or 2 mm (0.2 mV) in a precordial lead. If a pathologic cardiac problem exists, the ST segment elevation is often associated with other ECG changes, guiding the health care provider to a diagnosis.

24. B: Premature supraventricular beats appear as narrow QRS complexes that appear earlier than a normal sinus complex is expected. The P wave, QRS complex, and T wave are still present, indicating that the premature beat is supraventricular. When using automatic diagnostic reading devices, the device can be manually programmed to recognize premature supraventricular beats based on the timing between complexes.

25. D: The effective refractory period (ERP) acts as a protective mechanism for the heart by preventing irregular cellular depolarization. The refractory period limits the frequency of contractions that can be generated by the heart.

26. D: Atropine is the first drug of choice for symptomatic bradycardia. Dopamine and epinephrine are second-line agents for treating symptomatic bradycardia. Sotalol is a beta-blocker that would further slow the heart rate.

27. A: The PR interval represents speed of conduction from the atria to the ventricles. It may be shortened with increased heart rate, and lengthened with decreased heart rate. The speed of the heart rate is influenced by the sympathetic and parasympathetic nervous systems. This is the most common cause of spontaneous fluctuation in the PR interval. Certain medications and pathologies may also affect the PR interval, but often these changes are more consistent. Beta-blockers typically lengthen the PR interval. Individuals with an AV nodal bypass track typically have a shortened PR interval. An AV block may lengthen the PR interval.

28. C: A patient needs to achieve 85% to 90% of his or her age-predicted maximum heart rate during an exercise stress test in order for the test to be considered adequate for the detection of myocardial ischemia. If the patient is unable to exercise at this level, other forms of testing, such as pharmacologic stress testing, may need to be considered.

29. A: The right and left coronary arteries branch off from the root of the ascending aorta. The root of the ascending aorta refers to the beginning of the aorta, immediately after it exits the left ventricle.

30. B: Sinus tachycardia has a normal rhythm, but the rate is over 100 bpm. Normal sinus rhythm is 60 to 100 bpm. The P wave, QRS complex, and T wave are still present in sinus tachycardia, although they may be more difficult to differentiate if the rate is very high.

31. D: It can be very difficult to accurately diagnose myocardial ischemia on a Holter tracing if the patient has certain medical conditions or is on certain medications. Medical conditions that would interfere with the diagnosis include atrial fibrillation, atrial flutter, left bundle branch block, preexcitation, and serious ionic disorders. Medications that may interfere with diagnosis include digoxin, amiodarone, flecainide, antidepressants, and diuretics. In these cases, it is not advisable to give a diagnosis of myocardial ischemia based on Holter tracing findings. Beta-blockers are unlikely to interfere with diagnosing myocardial ischemia on the Holter tracing.

32. B: The cells of the SA node have the fastest rate of spontaneous depolarization in normal situations. Since the SA node depolarizes first, it establishes the heart rate and therefore is known as the cardiac pacemaker. Cells in the AV node, bundle branches, and Purkinje fibers have the potential to depolarize spontaneously, but would do so at a slower rate than the cells of the SA node, and would only do so under abnormal conditions.

33. A: The ventricular volume at the end of diastole is the preload. Stroke volume is the amount of blood that is pumped from the left ventricle in one contraction. Afterload is the end load against which the heart must overcome to eject blood. End-systolic volume is the ventricular volume after contraction.

34. C: An AV conduction problem is likely present if bradycardia is present during atrial fibrillation. On the tracing, fast irregular atrial activity would be present because of the atrial fibrillation along with a slow ventricular rhythm. The slow ventricular rhythm is either due to a transitory complete AV block or a permanent complete AV block, resulting in a junctional or ventricular escape rhythm. Junctional or ventricular escape rhythms would be slower than the normal heart rate.

35. A: An increased amount of poorly conducting tissue, such as fat, will lead to lower amplitude on the surface ECG. Any significant amount of poorly conducting tissue or fluid between the heart and chest wall may result in decreased amplitude of the ECG. Examples of other conditions that may lead to this finding include a pericardial effusion or emphysema.

36. C: The normal resting membrane potential for the majority of myocardial cells is between 80 and 95 mV. The cell interior is negative relative to the extracellular area. The resting potential is set by the balance between inward sodium and calcium currents and outward potassium currents.

37. C: Deoxygenated blood from the body is carried to the right atrium by the vena cava. It is then pumped to the lungs by the right ventricle, where it becomes oxygenated, and then returned to the left atrium. Oxygenated blood moves from the left atrium to the left ventricle and is then pumped to the body through the aorta.

38. B: Any electrical equipment should be treated with care in order to ensure the safety of the patient and the staff using the equipment. To avoid electric shock of a patient, there are several steps that must be taken, including ensuring that the chassis is grounded and making sure that the patient is not connected to a ground or to monitoring equipment that provides a direct connection to the ground. Line isolation transformers prevent a circuit from being completed by connection to ground, thereby reducing electrocution hazard.

39. A: QRS duration, QRS morphology, tachycardia speed, and tachycardia onset may be helpful in differentiating ventricular from supraventricular tachycardia. The wider the QRS, the more likely it is of ventricular origin, especially if it is greater than 140 msec. With ventricular tachycardia, a monomorphous morphology is more common. A slower tachycardia, with a heart rate between 100 and 140 bpm would more likely indicate ventricular origin. When the first complex is only very slightly premature, this indicates a ventricular origin.

40. C: The bundle of His contains specialized muscle fibers that play an important role in the conduction of electrical impulses through the heart. The bundle of His splits into the left and right bundle branches, which transmit the current to the left and right ventricles. The bundle branches eventually give rise to Purkinje fibers that distribute the impulse to the ventricular muscle.

41. A: Digitalis slows conduction through the AV node by increasing vagal tone. It is used for controlling the ventricular response in atrial fibrillation and atrial flutter and is also effective for the treatment of certain reentrant paroxysmal supraventricular tachycardias. However, digitalis toxicity can cause many types of arrhythmias. Frequent premature ventricular contractions are often the first sign of digitalis toxicity. The patient may develop ventricular tachycardia and then ventricular fibrillation if the digitalis toxicity is not recognized and treated.

42. C: Absolute contraindications to stress testing include acute pericarditis, acute myocarditis, suspected dissecting aneurysm, pulmonary embolism, symptomatic heart failure, ECG changes suggesting recent MI or severe ischemia, unstable angina, uncontrolled arrhythmias, and severe symptomatic aortic stenosis. Patients who are unable to exercise can do a nonexercise form of stress test. The ECG is more difficult to interpret in patients with a complete left bundle branch block and these patients may have to have modified forms of stress testing. One of the purposes of stress testing is to evaluate for coronary artery disease.

43. D: Skeletal muscle tremor can show up as an electrical artifact on ECG tracings. It classically looks like irregular, spiky oscillations of the baseline, and may mimic atrial fibrillation or other cardiac abnormalities. It is necessary to find out the cause of the tremor and to find a solution. If the patient is tense, provide reassurance and ask them to relax. If they are cold, ensure the room is warm and provide blankets. If they have Parkinson disease or another cause of tremor, move the limb electrodes closer to the torso or have the patient tuck their hands under their body.

44. C: Five or more electrodes are placed on the trunk for the purposes of ambulatory monitoring. Electrodes are not placed on the arms and legs because of the high probability of muscle artifact.

45. C: Showering and bathing should be avoided while the Holter monitor is in use, as these activities are likely to cause the electrodes to become dislodged. All other normal daily activities should be continued. The purpose of the Holter monitor is to catch abnormalities that occur during normal daily activities.

46. A: "A" describes the classic look of atrial flutter on ECG. This is often described as a "saw-tooth" pattern. Inverting the tracing may help you identify this abnormality. "B" describes what may be seen in a case of atrial fibrillation. "C" describes what is most likely sinus tachycardia. "D" describes ventricular flutter.

47. B: Certain cardiac cells spontaneously depolarize, which is referred to as automaticity. The depolarization of the cell leads to an action potential being formed. Spontaneously depolarizing cardiac cells, such as those in the SA node, have unstable resting potentials created by positive sodium and calcium ions flowing slowly and continuously into the cell while the cell is at rest. As a result of the inflow of positive ions, the cell slowly depolarizes until it reaches a point where it triggers a change in membrane permeability. This change allows for the positively charged ions (mainly sodium) to move more quickly into the cell, depolarizing it further until an action potential is produced. The plasma membranes of these cells have reduced permeability to potassium while at rest. The sympathetic and parasympathetic nervous systems can change the heart rate, but this is not considered "spontaneous" or "automaticity."

48. A: Antiarrhythmic agents are drugs that are used to suppress abnormal heart rhythms. Class I agents work by blocking sodium channels. Class II agents block sympathetic nervous system activity. Class III agents block potassium channels. Class IV agents block calcium channels.

49. D: When evaluating the ST segment it is important to note whether there is ST elevation or depression. The ST segment should be isoelectric, meaning that it should be at baseline. If the baseline is moving, it would be very difficult to know if the ST segment changes are present.

50. D: Dipyridamole, dobutamine, and adenosine are among the most widely used agents for stress testing. Regadenoson (Lexiscan) is another common agent used for this purpose. Pharmacologic agents are used to stress the heart when the patient is unable to exercise. Norepinephrine is not an agent that is used for pharmacologic stress testing.

How to Overcome Test Anxiety

Just the thought of taking a test is enough to make most people a little nervous. A test is an important event that can have a long-term impact on your future, so it's important to take it seriously and it's natural to feel anxious about performing well. But just because anxiety is normal, that doesn't mean that it's helpful in test taking, or that you should simply accept it as part of your life. Anxiety can have a variety of effects. These effects can be mild, like making you feel slightly nervous, or severe, like blocking your ability to focus or remember even a simple detail.

If you experience test anxiety—whether severe or mild—it's important to know how to beat it. To discover this, first you need to understand what causes test anxiety.

Causes of Test Anxiety

While we often think of anxiety as an uncontrollable emotional state, it can actually be caused by simple, practical things. One of the most common causes of test anxiety is that a person does not feel adequately prepared for their test. This feeling can be the result of many different issues such as poor study habits or lack of organization, but the most common culprit is time management. Starting to study too late, failing to organize your study time to cover all of the material, or being distracted while you study will mean that you're not well prepared for the test. This may lead to cramming the night before, which will cause you to be physically and mentally exhausted for the test. Poor time management also contributes to feelings of stress, fear, and hopelessness as you realize you are not well prepared but don't know what to do about it.

Other times, test anxiety is not related to your preparation for the test but comes from unresolved fear. This may be a past failure on a test, or poor performance on tests in general. It may come from comparing yourself to others who seem to be performing better or from the stress of living up to expectations. Anxiety may be driven by fears of the future—how failure on this test would affect your educational and career goals. These fears are often completely irrational, but they can still negatively impact your test performance.

> **Review Video: 3 Reasons You Have Test Anxiety**
> Visit mometrix.com/academy and enter code: 428468

Elements of Test Anxiety

As mentioned earlier, test anxiety is considered to be an emotional state, but it has physical and mental components as well. Sometimes you may not even realize that you are suffering from test anxiety until you notice the physical symptoms. These can include trembling hands, rapid heartbeat, sweating, nausea, and tense muscles. Extreme anxiety may lead to fainting or vomiting. Obviously, any of these symptoms can have a negative impact on testing. It is important to recognize them as soon as they begin to occur so that you can address the problem before it damages your performance.

> **Review Video: 3 Ways to Tell You Have Test Anxiety**
> Visit mometrix.com/academy and enter code: 927847

The mental components of test anxiety include trouble focusing and inability to remember learned information. During a test, your mind is on high alert, which can help you recall information and stay focused for an extended period of time. However, anxiety interferes with your mind's natural processes, causing you to blank out, even on the questions you know well. The strain of testing during anxiety makes it difficult to stay focused, especially on a test that may take several hours. Extreme anxiety can take a huge mental toll, making it difficult not only to recall test information but even to understand the test questions or pull your thoughts together.

> **Review Video: How Test Anxiety Affects Memory**
> Visit mometrix.com/academy and enter code: 609003

Effects of Test Anxiety

Test anxiety is like a disease—if left untreated, it will get progressively worse. Anxiety leads to poor performance, and this reinforces the feelings of fear and failure, which in turn lead to poor performances on subsequent tests. It can grow from a mild nervousness to a crippling condition. If allowed to progress, test anxiety can have a big impact on your schooling, and consequently on your future.

Test anxiety can spread to other parts of your life. Anxiety on tests can become anxiety in any stressful situation, and blanking on a test can turn into panicking in a job situation. But fortunately, you don't have to let anxiety rule your testing and determine your grades. There are a number of relatively simple steps you can take to move past anxiety and function normally on a test and in the rest of life.

> **Review Video: How Test Anxiety Impacts Your Grades**
> Visit mometrix.com/academy and enter code: 939819

Physical Steps for Beating Test Anxiety

While test anxiety is a serious problem, the good news is that it can be overcome. It doesn't have to control your ability to think and remember information. While it may take time, you can begin taking steps today to beat anxiety.

Just as your first hint that you may be struggling with anxiety comes from the physical symptoms, the first step to treating it is also physical. Rest is crucial for having a clear, strong mind. If you are tired, it is much easier to give in to anxiety. But if you establish good sleep habits, your body and mind will be ready to perform optimally, without the strain of exhaustion. Additionally, sleeping well helps you to retain information better, so you're more likely to recall the answers when you see the test questions.

Getting good sleep means more than going to bed on time. It's important to allow your brain time to relax. Take study breaks from time to time so it doesn't get overworked, and don't study right before bed. Take time to rest your mind before trying to rest your body, or you may find it difficult to fall asleep.

Review Video: The Importance of Sleep for Your Brain
Visit mometrix.com/academy and enter code: 319338

Along with sleep, other aspects of physical health are important in preparing for a test. Good nutrition is vital for good brain function. Sugary foods and drinks may give a burst of energy but this burst is followed by a crash, both physically and emotionally. Instead, fuel your body with protein and vitamin-rich foods.

Also, drink plenty of water. Dehydration can lead to headaches and exhaustion, especially if your brain is already under stress from the rigors of the test. Particularly if your test is a long one, drink water during the breaks. And if possible, take an energy-boosting snack to eat between sections.

Review Video: How Diet Can Affect your Mood
Visit mometrix.com/academy and enter code: 624317

Along with sleep and diet, a third important part of physical health is exercise. Maintaining a steady workout schedule is helpful, but even taking 5-minute study breaks to walk can help get your blood pumping faster and clear your head. Exercise also releases endorphins, which contribute to a positive feeling and can help combat test anxiety.

When you nurture your physical health, you are also contributing to your mental health. If your body is healthy, your mind is much more likely to be healthy as well. So take time to rest, nourish your body with healthy food and water, and get moving as much as possible. Taking these physical steps will make you stronger and more able to take the mental steps necessary to overcome test anxiety.

Mental Steps for Beating Test Anxiety

Working on the mental side of test anxiety can be more challenging, but as with the physical side, there are clear steps you can take to overcome it. As mentioned earlier, test anxiety often stems from lack of preparation, so the obvious solution is to prepare for the test. Effective studying may be the most important weapon you have for beating test anxiety, but you can and should employ several other mental tools to combat fear.

First, boost your confidence by reminding yourself of past success—tests or projects that you aced. If you're putting as much effort into preparing for this test as you did for those, there's no reason you should expect to fail here. Work hard to prepare; then trust your preparation.

Second, surround yourself with encouraging people. It can be helpful to find a study group, but be sure that the people you're around will encourage a positive attitude. If you spend time with others who are anxious or cynical, this will only contribute to your own anxiety. Look for others who are motivated to study hard from a desire to succeed, not from a fear of failure.

Third, reward yourself. A test is physically and mentally tiring, even without anxiety, and it can be helpful to have something to look forward to. Plan an activity following the test, regardless of the outcome, such as going to a movie or getting ice cream.

When you are taking the test, if you find yourself beginning to feel anxious, remind yourself that you know the material. Visualize successfully completing the test. Then take a few deep, relaxing breaths and return to it. Work through the questions carefully but with confidence, knowing that you are capable of succeeding.

Developing a healthy mental approach to test taking will also aid in other areas of life. Test anxiety affects more than just the actual test—it can be damaging to your mental health and even contribute to depression. It's important to beat test anxiety before it becomes a problem for more than testing.

> **Review Video: Test Anxiety and Depression**
> Visit mometrix.com/academy and enter code: 904704

Study Strategy

Being prepared for the test is necessary to combat anxiety, but what does being prepared look like? You may study for hours on end and still not feel prepared. What you need is a strategy for test prep. The next few pages outline our recommended steps to help you plan out and conquer the challenge of preparation.

STEP 1: SCOPE OUT THE TEST

Learn everything you can about the format (multiple choice, essay, etc.) and what will be on the test. Gather any study materials, course outlines, or sample exams that may be available. Not only will this help you to prepare, but knowing what to expect can help to alleviate test anxiety.

STEP 2: MAP OUT THE MATERIAL

Look through the textbook or study guide and make note of how many chapters or sections it has. Then divide these over the time you have. For example, if a book has 15 chapters and you have five days to study, you need to cover three chapters each day. Even better, if you have the time, leave an extra day at the end for overall review after you have gone through the material in depth.

If time is limited, you may need to prioritize the material. Look through it and make note of which sections you think you already have a good grasp on, and which need review. While you are studying, skim quickly through the familiar sections and take more time on the challenging parts. Write out your plan so you don't get lost as you go. Having a written plan also helps you feel more in control of the study, so anxiety is less likely to arise from feeling overwhelmed at the amount to cover.

STEP 3: GATHER YOUR TOOLS

Decide what study method works best for you. Do you prefer to highlight in the book as you study and then go back over the highlighted portions? Or do you type out notes of the important information? Or is it helpful to make flashcards that you can carry with you? Assemble the pens, index cards, highlighters, post-it notes, and any other materials you may need so you won't be distracted by getting up to find things while you study.

If you're having a hard time retaining the information or organizing your notes, experiment with different methods. For example, try color-coding by subject with colored pens, highlighters, or post-it notes. If you learn better by hearing, try recording yourself reading your notes so you can listen while in the car, working out, or simply sitting at your desk. Ask a friend to quiz you from your flashcards, or try teaching someone the material to solidify it in your mind.

STEP 4: CREATE YOUR ENVIRONMENT

It's important to avoid distractions while you study. This includes both the obvious distractions like visitors and the subtle distractions like an uncomfortable chair (or a too-comfortable couch that makes you want to fall asleep). Set up the best study environment possible: good lighting and a comfortable work area. If background music helps you focus, you may want to turn it on, but otherwise keep the room quiet. If you are using a computer to take notes, be sure you don't have any other windows open, especially applications like social media, games, or anything else that could distract you. Silence your phone and turn off notifications. Be sure to keep water close by so you stay hydrated while you study (but avoid unhealthy drinks and snacks).

Also, take into account the best time of day to study. Are you freshest first thing in the morning? Try to set aside some time then to work through the material. Is your mind clearer in the afternoon or evening? Schedule your study session then. Another method is to study at the same time of day that you will take the test, so that your brain gets used to working on the material at that time and will be ready to focus at test time.

STEP 5: STUDY!

Once you have done all the study preparation, it's time to settle into the actual studying. Sit down, take a few moments to settle your mind so you can focus, and begin to follow your study plan. Don't give in to distractions or let yourself procrastinate. This is your time to prepare so you'll be ready to fearlessly approach the test. Make the most of the time and stay focused.

Of course, you don't want to burn out. If you study too long you may find that you're not retaining the information very well. Take regular study breaks. For example, taking five minutes out of every hour to walk briskly, breathing deeply and swinging your arms, can help your mind stay fresh.

As you get to the end of each chapter or section, it's a good idea to do a quick review. Remind yourself of what you learned and work on any difficult parts. When you feel that you've mastered the material, move on to the next part. At the end of your study session, briefly skim through your notes again.

But while review is helpful, cramming last minute is NOT. If at all possible, work ahead so that you won't need to fit all your study into the last day. Cramming overloads your brain with more information than it can process and retain, and your tired mind may struggle to recall even previously learned information when it is overwhelmed with last-minute study. Also, the urgent nature of cramming and the stress placed on your brain contribute to anxiety. You'll be more likely to go to the test feeling unprepared and having trouble thinking clearly.

So don't cram, and don't stay up late before the test, even just to review your notes at a leisurely pace. Your brain needs rest more than it needs to go over the information again. In fact, plan to finish your studies by noon or early afternoon the day before the test. Give your brain the rest of the day to relax or focus on other things, and get a good night's sleep. Then you will be fresh for the test and better able to recall what you've studied.

STEP 6: TAKE A PRACTICE TEST

Many courses offer sample tests, either online or in the study materials. This is an excellent resource to check whether you have mastered the material, as well as to prepare for the test format and environment.

Check the test format ahead of time: the number of questions, the type (multiple choice, free response, etc.), and the time limit. Then create a plan for working through them. For example, if you have 30 minutes to take a 60-question test, your limit is 30 seconds per question. Spend less time on the questions you know well so that you can take more time on the difficult ones.

If you have time to take several practice tests, take the first one open book, with no time limit. Work through the questions at your own pace and make sure you fully understand them. Gradually work up to taking a test under test conditions: sit at a desk with all study materials put away and set a timer. Pace yourself to make sure you finish the test with time to spare and go back to check your answers if you have time.

After each test, check your answers. On the questions you missed, be sure you understand why you missed them. Did you misread the question (tests can use tricky wording)? Did you forget the information? Or was it something you hadn't learned? Go back and study any shaky areas that the practice tests reveal.

Taking these tests not only helps with your grade, but also aids in combating test anxiety. If you're already used to the test conditions, you're less likely to worry about it, and working through tests until you're scoring well gives you a confidence boost. Go through the practice tests until you feel comfortable, and then you can go into the test knowing that you're ready for it.

Test Tips

On test day, you should be confident, knowing that you've prepared well and are ready to answer the questions. But aside from preparation, there are several test day strategies you can employ to maximize your performance.

First, as stated before, get a good night's sleep the night before the test (and for several nights before that, if possible). Go into the test with a fresh, alert mind rather than staying up late to study.

Try not to change too much about your normal routine on the day of the test. It's important to eat a nutritious breakfast, but if you normally don't eat breakfast at all, consider eating just a protein bar. If you're a coffee drinker, go ahead and have your normal coffee. Just make sure you time it so that the caffeine doesn't wear off right in the middle of your test. Avoid sugary beverages, and drink enough water to stay hydrated but not so much that you need a restroom break 10 minutes into the test. If your test isn't first thing in the morning, consider going for a walk or doing a light workout before the test to get your blood flowing.

Allow yourself enough time to get ready, and leave for the test with plenty of time to spare so you won't have the anxiety of scrambling to arrive in time. Another reason to be early is to select a good seat. It's helpful to sit away from doors and windows, which can be distracting. Find a good seat, get out your supplies, and settle your mind before the test begins.

When the test begins, start by going over the instructions carefully, even if you already know what to expect. Make sure you avoid any careless mistakes by following the directions.

Then begin working through the questions, pacing yourself as you've practiced. If you're not sure on an answer, don't spend too much time on it, and don't let it shake your confidence. Either skip it and come back later, or eliminate as many wrong answers as possible and guess among the remaining ones. Don't dwell on these questions as you continue—put them out of your mind and focus on what lies ahead.

Be sure to read all of the answer choices, even if you're sure the first one is the right answer. Sometimes you'll find a better one if you keep reading. But don't second-guess yourself if you do immediately know the answer. Your gut instinct is usually right. Don't let test anxiety rob you of the information you know.

If you have time at the end of the test (and if the test format allows), go back and review your answers. Be cautious about changing any, since your first instinct tends to be correct, but make sure you didn't misread any of the questions or accidentally mark the wrong answer choice. Look over any you skipped and make an educated guess.

At the end, leave the test feeling confident. You've done your best, so don't waste time worrying about your performance or wishing you could change anything. Instead, celebrate the successful completion of this test. And finally, use this test to learn how to deal with anxiety even better next time.

> **Review Video: 5 Tips to Beat Test Anxiety**
> Visit mometrix.com/academy and enter code: 570656

Important Qualification

Not all anxiety is created equal. If your test anxiety is causing major issues in your life beyond the classroom or testing center, or if you are experiencing troubling physical symptoms related to your anxiety, it may be a sign of a serious physiological or psychological condition. If this sounds like your situation, we strongly encourage you to seek professional help.

Thank You

We at Mometrix would like to extend our heartfelt thanks to you, our friend and patron, for allowing us to play a part in your journey. It is a privilege to serve people from all walks of life who are unified in their commitment to building the best future they can for themselves.

The preparation you devote to these important testing milestones may be the most valuable educational opportunity you have for making a real difference in your life. We encourage you to put your heart into it—that feeling of succeeding, overcoming, and yes, conquering will be well worth the hours you've invested.

We want to hear your story, your struggles and your successes, and if you see any opportunities for us to improve our materials so we can help others even more effectively in the future, please share that with us as well. **The team at Mometrix would be absolutely thrilled to hear from you!** So please, send us an email (support@mometrix.com) and let's stay in touch.

> **If you'd like some additional help, check out these other resources we offer for your exam:**
> **http://MometrixFlashcards.com/CCT**

Additional Bonus Material

Due to our efforts to try to keep this book to a manageable length, we've created a link that will give you access to all of your additional bonus material.

**Please visit
https://www.mometrix.com/bonus948/cct to
access the information.**